Designing a Research Project

Ronald G. Marks, Ph.D.

Designing a Research Project

THE BASICS OF BIOMEDICAL RESEARCH METHODOLOGY

VNR VAN NOSTRAND REINHOLD COMPANY
New York

To my wife, Cindy

Designer: Rick Chafian
Editor: Edna Miller
Composition: Syntax International

Printed in the United States of America

2 3 4 5 6 7 8 9 10——86 85

Library of Congress Cataloging in Publication Data

Marks, Ronald G.
Designing a research project.

Includes index.
1. Medical research—Methodology. 2. Biological research—Methodology. 3. Research—Methodology. I. Title. [DNLM: 1. Research design. W 20.5 M346d]
R850.M29 610′.72 82-109
ISBN 0-534-97940-8 AACR2

Contents

Projects

Preface

Purpose of This Book

Any research effort in the biomedical and related sciences requires the consideration of certain fundamental concepts of research design. This is something that in my experience few research projects actually address. The purpose of this work is to identify and discuss each of these concepts.

Intended Audience

This book is for those getting started in research and in need of learning its basic steps. This group includes a broad cross section of researchers in the medical, dental, and related health research areas, as well as students, residents, and interns. Also, experienced researchers may find that they overlook certain fundamental concepts, especially sample size determination; they, too, should find this book useful. I have included numerous examples from medicine, dentistry, pharmacy, veterinary medicine, nursing, and related health professions to assist all these audiences.

How to Use This Book

This book is intended not only for the researcher designing a project but also as a reference for someone writing a grant proposal, doing research for a dissertation or a thesis, or doing research to be published as an article in a journal. The book is written so that the busy professional can use it as a self-instruction guide and move through the chapters at any pace. Most chapters are independent, providing easy access to each component of research design. The exceptions are Chapters 2 and 10. Chapter 2 gives the important definitions used throughout the book. Chapter 10 presents examples of sample size estimation after an introduction to the topic in Chapter 9, so Chapter 9 should be read before Chapter 10.

After completing this text, you will have had an *introduction* to the areas of research design that are important to understand as you carry out any research project. You must realize that there is much more to learn about each of the topics discussed. References are provided to supplement each topic.

A Note on Clinical Trials and Epidemiological Studies

You may find it interesting that the terms *clinical trials* and *epidemiological studies* are not mentioned in this book. The reason is that the design concepts discussed in this text are important in *all* types of research projects, including clinical trial studies, epidemiological studies, and sample surveys. However, the emphasis on each topic would differ in the various types of studies. I feel that an entire book is required to discuss either clinical trial studies or epidemiological studies adequately, but that any such book would incorporate the research design considerations discussed in this book.

Acknowledgments

I would like to thank Dr. James Boen and Dr. Virginia Clark for reading the original manuscript and providing many helpful comments.

To conclude, let me emphasize that this book is *not* meant to replace your professional statistician. It introduces the topics that you must discuss with a statistician when you are designing a research project. It will improve the communication between you and your statistician. Of course, if no professional statistical help is available, you should use this book as a self-instruction guide to assist in the proper design of your research project.

I believe that an understanding of the topics in this book can help a researcher become more productive and efficient and, at the same time, enjoy research more by having a better understanding of research design.

Ronald G. Marks

A Note to Course Instructors

Designing a Research Project has worked well as the first course in a two-semester sequence that I teach on research design and statistical analysis methods. The topics in this book are taught in a two-hour first-semester course. The topics taught in my second-semester three-hour course are covered in my book *Analyzing Research Data.* I find that students who are introduced to the topics in these two books become more interested in doing research and retain more interest after completing their first research projects. I believe they retain interest because they are more successful in their initial attempts at research, avoiding many of the pitfalls that first-time researchers encounter.

CHAPTER 1

Planning a Research Project

1.1 PURPOSE FOR THE BEGINNING RESEARCHER

If you are undertaking your first research project, you must consider the total planning effort required to guarantee the success of the project. The mental planning of any research project is at least as important as the physical collection of the data. This mental aspect deals with all the step-by-step planning that is required *before* the data collection can begin.

This planning involves choosing an appropriate design for the project. What data should be collected? How much? From whom? In planning, you also determine how the data will be processed and managed, and you decide on the appropriate statistical analysis of the data. If you do not plan carefully before you start collecting data, the result may be that you cannot achieve the research objective because of an inappropriate design.

This book will provide you, the beginning researcher, with the basic planning steps required in any research project. It will help you to avoid the mistakes made through inappropriate planning and to achieve a successful research project in the first attempt. Finally, you will have a better understanding of the topics with which a statistician can assist, and your communication with your statistician will be improved.

1.2 PURPOSE FOR THE EXPERIENCED RESEARCHER

As an experienced researcher, you already know many of the concepts discussed here. Most experienced researchers, however, will learn some new and useful information. For example, Chapters 9 and 10, dealing with the determination of the needed sample size for a research project to achieve its stated objective, provide information that still is overlooked by most researchers but is essential for anyone planning to submit a grant proposal. If a statistician helps with your sample size estimation, the information he or she will need from you is illustrated in these chapters.

If you are an experienced researcher, you can proceed immediately to the chapters of interest without having to read all the preceding chapters. The only exceptions are Chapters 2 and 10. Chapter 2 presents the basic, important terms for all research projects. Each succeeding chapter uses this terminology, so you should read Chapter 2 before any other chapters.

Chapters 9 and 10 both deal with sample size estimation. You should read the basic concepts in Chapter 9 before proceeding to the examples in Chapter 10.

1.3 WHAT YOU WILL LEARN ABOUT RESEARCH METHODOLOGY

Whether you are a beginning or an experienced researcher, this book should benefit you by improving your research techniques. It certainly will not teach you all there is to know about research methodology, but it will provide a foundation for the successful completion of any research project, regardless of its size or complexity. After learning these basics, you can go on to learn more about the particular areas that apply to your individual efforts and build on your research methodology foundation.

1.4 PROBLEMS FROM POOR PLANNING

To see some common types of errors that are committed in research projects because of inadequate planning before the data collection begins, let us look at a few examples.

1.4.1 Example: Improper Assignment of Subjects to Treatments

A researcher wishes to compare the effectiveness of a nitroglycerin paste to a standard nitroglycerin pill in the treatment of patients with angina pectoris. The results of the research project indicate that the new paste is not effective in comparison with the standard pill. More people receiving the paste die, and also they die earlier than do people receiving the standard pill. Upon being questioned, the researcher reveals that the assignment of patients to treatment groups was not random. Since the researcher believed the paste to be superior to the standard pill, the most seriously ill patients were assigned to receive the paste treatment. This decision was an appropriate moral one, but it completely invalidated any comparison of the two treatments. A more scientific assignment of patients to the two groups is essential for comparison of the effectiveness of the treatments.

This researcher failed to consider a scientific method for assigning patients to each treatment group in such a way as to 1) allow a comparison of the two treatments and 2) provide each patient with the best possible medical care. He or she also failed to consider adequately the consequences of using the chosen assignment scheme. This researcher avoided a key mental point in planning the research project, and the result was a project that yielded no valid results.

1.4.2 Example: Variability Among Subjects

The Environmental Protection Agency (EPA) is asked by a utility company for permission to burn a fuel that releases more SO_2 into the air than does their current fuel. The EPA believes that this change will have an impact on breathing for people near this utility, so a researcher is given a grant to evaluate this claim. People involved in the study breathe either normal air or air plus SO_2, and their breathing is monitored and measured. Although the researcher expects the breathing to be hindered by the SO_2, the analysis of the data yields no important differences. A careful review of the research project reveals that there is a large difference among people in their breathing ability, regardless of what is added to the air. This variability among people is enough to cause the comparison of normal air to SO_2 to be clouded. The researcher should have considered this problem *before* performing the research project. Then alternative design considerations for the project, such as having each person studied under *both* breathing conditions at different times or increasing the sample size, could have been presented and would have resolved this problem.

If such other designs are not considered feasible, the researcher should decide whether it is worth spending the time and money to perform this project if the research objective probably will not be attained.

This researcher perceived a serious shortcoming in the experimental design, but only *after* the conclusion of the project. As a result, a great physical and financial effort was expended and the results are not what the researcher hoped to show. An important design consideration was overlooked before the project was begun.

1.4.3 Example: Optimistic Schedule for Study Completion

Another researcher plans to evaluate a drug developed for patients who have had coronary bypass surgery. The researcher has four months (October through January) to carry out this project before leaving this position. Because the hospital performs two to three of these operations each week and about half the patients receiving this surgery will be eligible for this study, the researcher feels that it will be possible to include about 30 people in the study during the three months of data collection. The remaining month will be spent in initial preparation for the project and in analysis of the final results.

One major task in preparation for this project is to receive approval from the local institutional review board (IRB). Problems in acquiring this approval because of a poorly worded consent form delay the start of the study until mid-November. The number of operations performed from mid-November until the end of the year drop off greatly because of the holidays. During this time, only emergency operations are performed; and because emergency operations cannot be included in this study, the researcher cannot begin data collection until January. By the end of January, 10 patients have been studied and the researcher has not yet performed the data analysis.

Although this researcher originally considered how large a sample could be obtained, time was not budgeted for unforeseen delays and holiday periods. Again, this project does not achieve its expectations because of a mental error. Had the researcher considered these problems before the project began, it might have been possible to consider alternative plans to get around these problems or to decide that the project was not worth beginning.

1.4.4 Example: Poor Data Management

Another researcher has a multiyear grant that involves collecting a large amount of data. As the data are collected, they are placed on computer cards, but no single person is responsible for managing the data. After a few years, when the time comes to report the results to the granting agency, the researcher realizes that some data cannot be found, that the data were not stored uniformly over the years, and that no one on the current staff is familiar with all the transitions made in the data over the years. Moreover, since no one was responsible for data storage and handling, there is no one to whom the researcher may look for solutions to these problems. The result is that the researcher cannot produce the desired information for the granting agency. Hence, the grant is not renewed. Years of hard work led to incomplete results because of the omission of a very important part of the research project, data management.

This researcher failed at the beginning of the research project to provide adequately for the management and analysis of the data. Although the researcher may have had no expertise to handle this important part of the research project directly, he or she should have assumed ultimate responsibility for seeing that this job was performed. As in the first three examples, the mental aspect of planning the entire research project was not completely carried out.

1.5 THE VALUE OF MENTAL PLANNING

Each of these examples illustrates a different mental error that is common in biomedical research projects. These errors result from lack of planning by the researcher. They can be avoided if they are considered before the data collection begins, and they can ruin a project if they are overlooked. The result will be a waste of the researcher's time and money, since the experimental objective will not be attained. **The success of a research project depends on how**

well thought out the project is and on how potential problems have been identified and resolved before the data collection begins. By reading this text and discussing your planned research project with a statistician, if available, you can go a long way toward minimizing the problems that will be encountered.

A problem that researchers face is that many courses offered to them contain more emphasis on the computational aspects of performing statistical analyses than on design considerations. More attention should be paid to deciding *which* analysis should be performed than to *how* to compute it. Desk-top calculators and packaged computer programs today can perform all the necessary data analysis for us. Therefore, a researcher needs to concentrate on how to choose the best design and which analysis should be used on the collected data. This statement is true whether the researcher is planning the research project for a grant proposal, a thesis or dissertation, or independent research to be published in a scientific journal.

1.6 SPECIFIC AIMS OF THIS BOOK

The objective of this book is to provide a working knowledge of the basic rules to follow in research. Specifically, the book is designed to aid you in the following areas:

1. choosing an efficient research design
2. handling data appropriately for processing and data management
3. evaluating the research of others
4. weighting practical constraints against scientific needs

1.7 STRUCTURE OF THIS BOOK

Data collection in a research project should not begin until the following questions have been satisfactorily answered.

1. What is the overall objective of the research project?
2. What type of data will be collected?
3. What selection process will be used in the choice of subjects for the project?
4. If various treatments are to be compared, can and should subjects receive more than one treatment?
5. How should the subjects be assigned to the various treatments?
6. How many subjects should be included in the project?
7. What will be done to put the data in a form suitable for analysis?
8. What is an appropriate statistical technique to use in data analysis?

The above questions all reflect mental steps that you must take before ever beginning to collect data. This volume provides a detailed look at each of the first seven questions listed above. These chapters deal with *scientific* as well as *practical* considerations. They present information that would have helped the researcher avoid the errors made in the first three examples we saw earlier.

Volume II discusses rules for choosing the appropriate statistical analyses of the data for your own project. References are provided for the researcher who wishes to learn more about the computational aspects of the various analyses. The analyses are representative of those commonly used with biomedical data. They do *not* represent all possible analyses, and you should not force your data into one of them if it does not seem totally appropriate. Instead, you should consult a statistician or someone who can determine the appropriate analysis for your project.

CHAPTER 2

Step One: Determining the Objective and Identifying Research Components

2.1 INTRODUCTION

The first step in a research project is to state its objective clearly. You must choose a project that will be meaningful when completed and also one that can be accomplished practically. One means of evaluating the objective is through a literature review. This important process establishes the validity and potential of a research project. A comprehensive review provides an outline of previous research on your topic and should show the possible benefits of the proposed research. Ideas on carrying out literature reviews vary among disciplines, so no attempt will be made here to describe a unique method. Do not, however, underestimate its importance. A literature review is vital.

In this chapter, we shall see how to determine the overall objective of the research and relate the objective to the research process to be performed.

2.2 STATING YOUR OBJECTIVE

Have you ever read a journal article and afterwards wondered what the researcher was trying to prove? Or has someone ever asked you during the course of a research project what you were trying to prove and you had to think a while before being able to answer? In either case, the researcher does not clearly understand the objective of the project and, hence, cannot know that the chosen design is the best and most efficient way to achieve that objective. On the other hand, a concise statement of the objective shows that the researcher has a clear understanding of the purpose of the research project.

Regardless of the complexity and size of the research project, the overall objective should be stated as simply as possible. For example, the objective "to study the relationship of type of antidiarrheic drug (Drug A and Drug B), nutrition plan (Plan X and Plan Y), and length of hospitalization on the initial weight loss of patients having gastric partition surgery" is stated clearly and concisely.

Another clearly stated objective is "to compare two drugs for treating epilepsy (new Drug X versus standard Drug Y) to determine whether the rate of epileptic seizures is lower for people using one of these drugs." Also, "to evaluate a newly developed educational procedure to determine whether grade school children who are prejudiced toward physically handicapped children have improved attitudes after this education" provides others with a clear picture of the objective of the researcher's project.

You probably already have performed some research or are planning to in the near future. Can you put the overall objective of your research project in a concise statement?

2.3 RELATING THE OBJECTIVE TO THE RESEARCH PROCESS

A problem arises in many research projects when the researcher is not quantitatively oriented. This researcher has a difficult time relating the practical, stated objective to the actual research process. For example, suppose the objective of a research project is "to evaluate Vaccines A and B to determine whether the incidence rate of a flu virus is lower in children receiving one of these vaccines." In this project we are interested in the *children* and in determining which *vaccine* is better at preventing *flu*. This is our practical concern. However, to determine the answer to this objective, we shall have to collect some type of *data* and perform some *statistical analysis* to determine which vaccine is better. To succeed, we must be able to consider the numerical (data) aspects of the research project. Before beginning our design, we must develop some terms that will link the practical statement of the research objective to the research process that will be carried out to achieve this objective. You must identify the following terms for your own project if you are to develop the best and most efficient design and to choose the correct statistical data analysis.

2.4 BASIC TERMINOLOGY

2.4.1 Experimental Unit and Response Variable

The collection of data in a research project involves the observation of some response (or responses) on each of a group of objects. Each object studied in the project is called an **experimental unit.** The most common types of experimental units studied are people and animals. However, bacterial cultures, vials of drugs, and medical charts all are examples of possible experimental units.

The observation relevant to the physical phenomenon being studied on the experimental unit is called the **response variable.** For example, if we are studying hypertension in adults, each person studied is an experimental unit, and the blood pressure observations (systolic and diastolic) for each person are the response variables related to hypertension. If we are studying glaucoma in beagles, each beagle is an experimental unit. Since intraocular pressure (IOP) in the eye is used to measure glaucoma, IOP is the response variable. Note that more than one response variable may be measured on each experimental unit. In the hypertension example, both systolic and diastolic pressure were measured. Another term for response variable is **dependent variable** or **outcome.**

2.4.2 Universe and Population

Of practical interest to the researcher is the entire collection of experimental units that exist. If elderly people, defined as those over 65 years of age, are being studied, then the researcher is interested in the group of all elderly people. If adolescents with diabetes are being studied, the researcher is interested in the group of all diabetic adolescents. From the researcher's viewpoint, the collection of all the experimental units is referred to as the population of interest, and the objective of the project is stated in terms of this population.

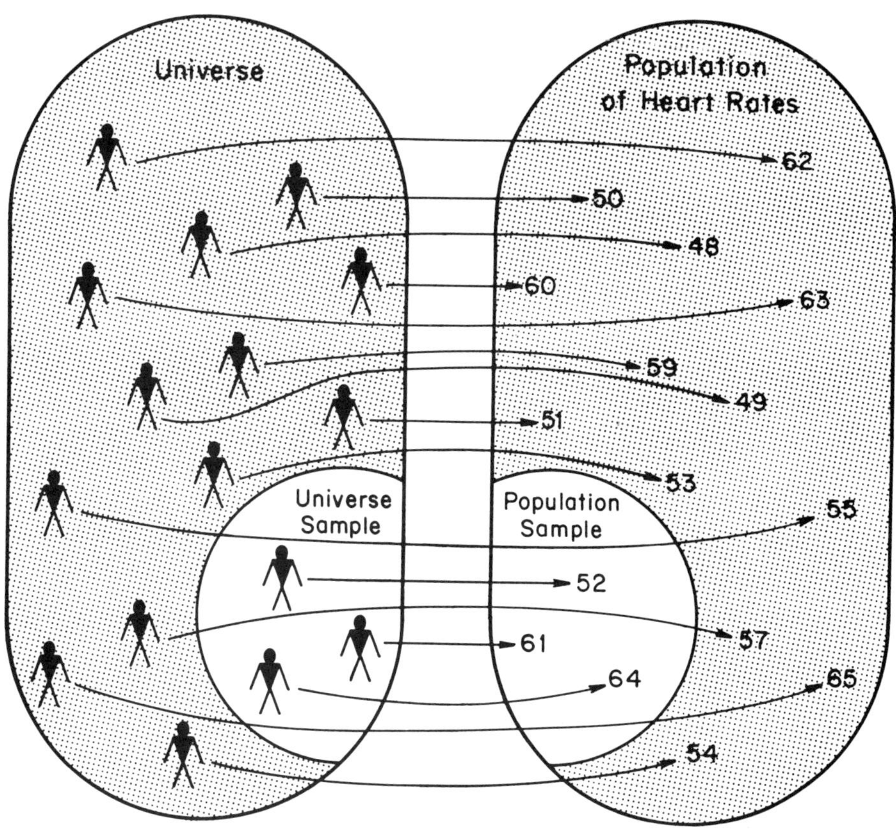

Figure 2.1 Universe and population.

On the other hand, for the purposes of data collection, the population of interest is the collection of measurements of the response variables on all the experimental units. Therefore, from a practical viewpoint, the population of interest is the collection of all experimental units, while from a research process point of view, the population of interest is the collection of the response variable measurements from all experimental units. Confusion sometimes exists in discussion between researchers because population can be thought of in two different ways. The confusion becomes especially apparent in discussions between biomedical researchers and data analysts.

Here, we shall refer to the practical population (people, dogs, medical charts, or all experimental units) as the **universe** and to the collection of the response variable measurements on each experimental unit as the **population.** For example, in the hypertension study, the collection of all people is the universe and the collection of blood pressures on all the people is the population. In the glaucoma example, the collection of all beagles is the universe and the collection of IOPs from all beagles is the population. Note that the universe and hence, the population, may be either finite or infinite in size.

2.4.3 Universe Sample and Population Sample

Because the entire universe cannot be studied, a representative selection of experimental units should be chosen and the response variable measured on those experimental units. The collection of the experimental units included in the study will be called the **universe sample** (henceforth, denoted **U-sample**) and the response variable measurements on those experimental units shall be the **population sample** (denoted **P-sample**). (See Figure 2.1.) In the hypertension example, the people included in the study are the U-sample, and their blood pressure measurements are the P-sample.

These terms define the objects studied in the project and the measurements being taken that describe the phenomenon under study. There are other terms to be defined, but first we must distinguish between two types of research projects: **experimental studies** and **observational studies.**

2.5 EXPERIMENTAL STUDIES

Here is an example of an experimental research project.

Project 2.1 A comparison of two dental sealants

A dental researcher wishes to compare a newly developed tooth sealant to an existing commercial brand for its ability to prevent caries in elementary school children. Students will be selected to participate in the study and will be assigned to one of the two competing sealants. The students will receive the sealant and will be studied every six months for two years to document their caries experience. At that time, the researcher can determine whether or not the new sealant is superior to the existing one in the prevention of caries. In this study, the researcher has control over who enters the study because he or she can establish the criteria necessary for participation. For example, the researcher may decide to study only first and second graders, because their first molars would be erupting and could be sealed before becoming carious. Or, he or she may decide to study fifth and sixth graders whose premolars would be erupting. The study will include only children with at least one contralateral pair of caries-free teeth, and the reason for this will be shown in a later chapter. The researcher may also decide to limit the study to children from middle class families or to children who see their dentists regularly, so that the study groups will be relatively homogeneous and provide the fairest comparison of the two sealants.

In addition, the researcher controls the assignment of sealants to participants in the study. This control allows the researcher to assign the brands equally over age groups, between males and females, and between dental hygiene groups (e.g., good and poor dental hygiene), which leads to a balanced assignment of sealant brands. This approach also will insure the researcher of the fairest comparison of the two sealants.

Let us now evaluate the important terms for this study and then point out what makes it an experimental study. The objective of this project is **to determine whether a new tooth sealant (Brand A) is superior to an existing sealant (Brand B) in preventing caries.** For this project, the researcher will define

Universe	All elementary school children with at least one contralateral pair of caries-free teeth
Experimental unit	Each child in the above defined universe
Response variable	The number of caries after two years of the sealant
Population	The collection of cavity counts for all children in the universe
U-sample	The collection of children included in the study
P-sample	The collection of cavity counts on the children in the study

2.5.1 Factors

In this project, the researcher wishes to compare two tooth sealants on the prevention of caries. The two brands can be thought of as different types of treatment to be evaluated. Many research problems are similar to this example except that the types of treatment to be evaluated may instead be three different types of surgery (Surgeries A, B, and C), two diets (Diets X and Y), four cancer drugs (Drugs A, B, C, and D), or three dosages of a particular drug (5 cc, 10 cc, 15 cc). The treatment in each case will be defined as a **factor,** and the various settings of the factor will be denoted as their **levels.** (A factor also is called an **independent variable.**) An experimental study always will include at least one factor to be evaluated, and any number of factors may be present. The common denominator of experimental studies is that the primary factor to be evaluated will have its various levels assigned to the experimental units by the researcher. Thus, we shall define an **experimental factor** as one in which the researcher is responsible for assigning the levels to the experimental units.

Each experimental factor will have at least two levels and may have more than that. All experimental factors may be further classified as one of two types. **Qualitative factors** are factors in which the levels are categorical in nature (such as sealant brand or type of surgery or diet or drug). **Quantitative factors** are factors in which the levels are numerical in nature (such as 5 cc, 10 cc, 15 cc of a drug).

One other type of factor may exist in an experimental research project. In the sealant example, the researcher is concerned about assigning an equal proportion of each sealant brand across age groups, between males and females, and between the two dental hygiene groups. This concern exists because younger children may have a different caries rate from that of older children. Also, girls may have a different caries rate from boys, and children with poor dental hygiene may have a different caries rate from children with good dental hygiene. Thus, the researcher must be sure that each brand is tried equally in these groups.

In this project, age, sex, and dental hygiene are extraneous factors. **Extraneous factors** are those that are not of real interest to us but may affect the response variable. Thus, we must try to control for extraneous factors in an experimental study by assigning each level of the experimental factor an equal number of times across the levels of the extraneous factors.

The similarity of all experimental studies is that the researcher has complete control over assigning the levels of the experimental factors to the experimental units. Also, if any extraneous factors are present, the researcher can balance out their effects on the response variable through an appropriate assignment of factor levels. Note that the researcher does not have control over the assignment of levels of any extraneous factor to the experimental unit, because these levels already exist. Chapter 11 will present techniques for controlling extraneous factors and assigning levels of factors to experimental units.

Let us now contrast an experimental study with an observational study.

2.6 OBSERVATIONAL STUDIES

An example of an observational study would be the following.

Project 2.2 A study of factors related to the occurrence of brucellosis in florida dairy cattle

Brucellosis is a reproductive disease in cattle and is very prevalent in some areas in the South. Even cattle coming from areas where brucellosis has been eradicated may become exposed to the disease during transit when housed with cattle from other areas. Hence, it would be desirable to vaccinate all cattle coming into Florida, preferably at around six to eight months of age.

There are a number of factors to evaluate for the prevention of brucellosis. Various drugs can be used for vaccination, a different number of shots can be used on various herds, the age of the animal when the first shot is administered can differ, and the location of the shots on the animal's body can vary. Thus, the objective of this research project is **to determine whether an animal's vaccination history is related to whether or not brucellosis occurs.** The terms for this project are as follows.

Universe	All cattle raised in the South and susceptible to brucellosis
Experimental unit	Each cow in the universe
Response variable	Either *yes* (brucellosis is present) or *no* (no brucellosis is present)
Population	The collection of *yes* and *no* measurements for all the cattle in the universe
U-sample	The collection of all cattle included in the study
P-sample	The collection of *yes* and *no* measurements for all the cattle in the study

This study has factors to be evaluated, just as did the experimental study.

QUALITATIVE FACTORS

Factor 1: Type of vaccination
Level 1: None
Level 2: Vaccine A
Level 3: Vaccine B
Level 4: Vaccine C

Factor 2: Location of shot
Level 1: Subcutaneous (beneath the skin)
Level 2: Intradermal (into the skin)
Level 3: Conjunctival sac (in eye)

QUANTITATIVE FACTORS

Factor 3: Number of shots

Factor 4: Age at which first shot is given

Note that each quantitative factor can have a large number of levels, because the researcher has no control over how many shots are given or when they are given. The same could be true for Factor 1 if there are many vaccines that could be administered. The common thread of all observational studies is that the researcher has no control over the assignment of factor levels to experimental units or even over the number of levels that may occur. Let us then define an **observational factor** as one in which the researcher merely observes which level is present for an experimental unit. However, the objective is the same as that in experimental studies: to evaluate the relationship between various factors and a set of response variables.

Sometimes a researcher is interested in comparing subgroups of experimental units on some response variable rather than in evaluating a set of treatments on a response variable. For example, this researcher may wish to compare different breeds of cows, such as Holstein, Guernsey, and Jersey, for the prevalence of brucellosis. In many studies, researchers wish to evaluate the influence of race or sex on some response variable. Breed of cow, race, sex, and other classifying characteristics also are factors, and each of their categories is a level. Thus, a factor can be a set of treatments of some type or various groupings of the experimental units to compare on some response variable.

Extraneous factors exist in observational studies and pose more of a problem than they do in experimental studies because of the researcher's lack of control in balancing over these levels. For example, if geographic location in the South were an extraneous factor (that is, if cows in one location are more susceptible to brucellosis than are cows in a different location), the researcher could not balance factors 1 through 4 in each geographic location. It is conceivable that all cattle in one area were not vaccinated, or that if they were vaccinated, they all received the same drug. If this situation occurs, geographic location is said to be **confounded** with type of vaccine. The reason is that if brucellosis is more prevalent in these animals than in others, it is not known whether this fact results from geographic location or from type of vaccine (or even from some other unknown factor). The researcher cannot evaluate for a vaccine difference; and hence, information is lost. Thus, observational studies are characterized by the fact that levels of all factors are observed rather than assigned to experimental units.

Some studies contain both experimental and observational factors. As long as one experimental factor is present in the study, the study is experimental. Thus, a study is observational only if all factors are observational.

2.7 EXPERIMENTAL VERSUS OBSERVATIONAL STUDIES

In many research projects, the researcher does not have a choice between these types of studies because only an observational study is possible. However, if one is considering an experimental study, then its advantages and disadvantages should be compared to those of an observational study.

An experimental study generally is more expensive to perform than is a corresponding observational study. Choosing the experimental units is more expensive (that is, time consuming) in an experimental study because of advertising costs and controls imposed for inclusion in the study. Data collection also is generally more expensive, because people (as experimental units) usually are required to come to you. This arrangement often requires some sort of compensation. Also, time can be wasted when subjects do not keep appointments. If animals are used as the experimental units, their initial cost and boarding expenses must be covered. If some product is being compared to other commercially available products, the cost of purchasing these products must be considered in an experimental study.

Let us review the sealant study as an example. If both sealant brands are available commercially, many more responses can be obtained for the same cost through questionnaire mailings, telephone interviews, or interviews in the dentist's office. In this case the researcher is going to the people, getting instant responses, and being less restrictive as to who enters the study. (Dental hygiene could not be evaluated over the telephone.) Thus, observational studies usually can provide more data than can an experimental study.

Experimental studies, however, tend to provide "cleaner" results than do observational studies—that is, the results may be more acceptable and receive less criticism. This quality results from the control of extraneous factors. Experimental studies provide fewer data because more emphasis is placed on eliminating the influence of extraneous factors on the results. If the sealant study is done as an observational study, the researcher cannot be sure that the extraneous factors of age, sex, and dental hygiene are balanced over all brands. The hope is that the larger sample will lead to this balance, but the researcher cannot guarantee it.

Thus, it is up to the researcher to consider both types of studies (if both are feasible) and choose the one that will be most *practical* and *relevant* for achievement of the research objective.

You can gain experience in evaluating these types of studies by reading the examples in the following chapters.

2.8 PROSPECTIVE VERSUS RETROSPECTIVE STUDIES

One more distinction should be made between two types of studies. All studies are classified as either **prospective** or **retrospective.** A prospective study is one in which the researcher is planning to measure the response variable on each experimental unit at some future time. If the study is experimental, first the experimental units will be selected; then factor levels will be assigned; and finally, the response variable will be measured at some future time. If the study is observational, the researcher will first choose the experimental units and then observe the factor levels for each experimental unit. At some future time, the response variable measurement will be obtained. By their very nature, all experimental studies are prospective.

2.8.1 Types of Retrospective Studies

There are two general types of retrospective studies. First, in a **case-control study,** a group of experimental units with a particular response variable measurement (usually representing the presence of some disease state) is chosen for the study. Then, a control group, having a different response variable measurement (usually free of disease) also is chosen for the study. Then, by either a retrospective review of records or an interview with participants, the researcher can establish for each experimental unit the level that existed for the factor (or factors) of interest. The researcher then can compare the two groups, determined by the response variable measurement, to see whether the sets of factor levels are similar or different. If potential extraneous factors are identified, the control group can be chosen to match the first group on those factors. This procedure reduces the chances of the extraneous factors influencing the analysis. We shall say more about this matching procedure in Chapter 7.

In a **cross-sectional survey,** experimental units are chosen for the study and then the factor levels and response variable measurements are observed. In this type of retrospective study, it often is difficult to control for extraneous factors because the researcher is assessing the data at one particular time and has less ability to match on extraneous factors as the data are being collected.

We can compare a prospective study, a case-control study, and a cross-sectional survey on the basis of the time at which they occur. In a cross-sectional survey, both the factor levels and the response variable measurements are measured at a single point in time. In a case-control study, we determine the response variable measurement at the present time and the factor levels by going back in time to some predetermined point. In a prospective study, also called a **cohort study,** the factor levels are established for the present time and the response variable measurement is observed at some predetermined future point in time. An excellent discussion of each of these types of studies can be found in references 1 and 3 through 5.

2.8.2 Example: Prospective Study, Case-Control Study, and Cross-Sectional Survey

A research objective that has received a great deal of attention over the last 30 years is to determine whether or not a relationship exists between smoking history and the occurrence of lung cancer. Although this approach is highly unlikely, a researcher could decide to choose a group of nonsmokers, free of cancer, and assign half to a smoking group and the remaining half to a non-smoking group. At some later point in time, such as 10 years, the researcher could note for each person the response variable, which is whether or not lung cancer is present. This study would be an example of an experimental, prospective study. A more realistic approach for this type of study would be to choose a group of people free of cancer to participate in this study and merely to note their smoking history, instead of trying to influence that decision. Then, at some future time, the researcher could note whether or not lung cancer is present. This study would be an observational, prospective study.

If, on the other hand, the researcher chooses a group of people from a cancer clinic who have lung cancer and compares their smoking histories to those of a control group that is free of lung cancer, the study would be a case-control study and would be retrospective. Finally, if the researcher were to choose a group of people and determine at this time their individual smoking histories and whether or not they have lung cancer, the study would be classified as a cross-sectional study and would be retrospective. The key to whether a study is prospective or retrospective is whether the response variable measurement exists when the factor levels are observed or whether it will be obtained at some future time.

Note that in a cross-sectional survey, a cause and effect relationship cannot be established, because the factor level and response variable measurement are being measured simultaneously. In a prospective or case-control study, it is possible to determine a cause and effect relationship if potential extraneous factors are identified and controlled for, and if all other appropriate design considerations are made so that the results will be valid to extrapolate to the entire universe.

For more information on prospective and retrospective studies, see references 1 through 3.

2.9 PARAMETERS AND STATISTICS

In Chapter 4, we shall see that there are four types of response variables, both numerical and categorical. For each type of response variable, we must be able to describe the entire collection of response variable measurements, which is the population. A **parameter** is a single number used to describe a population of response variable measurements. Different parameters exist for the various types of response variables, and the research hypotheses to be studied often are stated in terms of the appropriate population parameter. The most commonly used parameters will be introduced in Chapter 4 after the different types of response variables are introduced.

The P-sample is a subset of the population of response variable measurements, and a number is needed to describe the P-sample. A **statistic** is a single number used to describe the collection of response variable measurements in a P-sample. The most commonly used statistics also will be introduced in Chapter 4, and their relationship to population parameters will be explained then.

The computed statistics are used to make inferences about the population parameter and, hence, answer the stated research hypothesis. More specific information on population parameters and P-sample statistics will be provided in future chapters.

2.10 LINKING THE RESEARCH COMPONENTS

To relate the *practical objective* of a research project to the *research process*, you first must be able to identify the terms we have discussed for your project. You will see as we go on that the decisions made will be determined from a knowledge of these terms. Therefore, the terms will provide the link between the practical objective and the research hypotheses. Good sources for more information on establishing the objective of the research are references 2, 4, and 5.

2.11 THE RESEARCH GOAL

You should always keep in mind the following goal of your research. The objective of any research project is to make some statement (inference, conclusion, decision) about a universe and the factors affecting that universe. To accomplish this goal, you record measurements (response variable) on a representative group (U-sample) from the universe. The collection of these measurements (P-sample) then is used to reach conclusions for the complete collection of measurements (population). You then relate the conclusion concerning the population to the universe of interest.

I have found it helpful to state the research objective in general terms as follows:

> To study (or determine or evaluate) the relationship between *list of factors* and *list of response variables* on *universe*.

This simple statement of the research objective defines and distinguishes between the factors and response variables included in the study, as well as defining the universe. We can thus restate some of the objectives we stated earlier: "To study the relationship between type of drug given and the epileptic seizure rate on the mentally retarded" and "to evaluate the relationship between type of educational procedure provided and the attitude of grade school children toward physically handicapped children."

Note that the terms *effect* and *influence* are not used in the statement of the research objective, because a single research project seldom can establish a cause and effect relationship. Numerous studies done over a period of time that eliminate all extraneous factors and biases are essential to establish a cause and effect relationship between sets of factors and response variables. An example would be the many studies performed and replicated to corroborate results before scientists became convinced that smoking causes cancer.

Each research objective in this book can be stated in this format. You may find it helpful to rewrite research objectives using this format to clarify the purpose of your study.

At the beginning of your study, you should state your specific objective and refer to it occasionally to be sure that you are proceeding toward that objective and have not become sidetracked toward another goal.

2.12 DEFINITIONS

The next chapter will present examples that illustrate the use of these terms in relation to the stated objective of the research project. Also, examples will be presented throughout the text, and in each example, these terms will be defined clearly so that they will become very familiar to you. Before going to the next chapter, let us provide a formal definition for each of the terms that have just been introduced.

Universe	The total collection of objects (people, animals, bacterial cultures, medical charts) that are of interest in the project
Experimental unit	Each individual object in the universe
Response variable (or dependent variable)	The observation or measurement that records the state of the experimental unit for the phenomenon being studied
Population	The collection of response variable measurements on all experimental units in the universe
U-sample	The group of experimental units included in the study
P-sample	The collection of response variable measurements from the U-sample
Factor (or independent variable)	A set of treatments or some other effect that is to be evaluated by the research work (type of diet, dose of drug); or groupings of experimental units into subsets of the universe for comparison (such as sex, age, or race)
Level of a factor	Each possible setting of a factor (Diet X and Diet Y; 5 cc, 10 cc, and 15 cc, of a drug; male and female)

Factors can be classified as follows:

Qualitative factor	One that has levels that are categorical (e.g., type of drug, type of surgery, type of birth control, sex)
Quantitative factor	One that has numerical levels (e.g., dose of drug, time spent in therapy, age)
Extraneous factor	A factor that is not of primary interest to the researcher but may have an effect on the response variable. It may be either qualitative or quantitative.

Factors also can be classified as follows:

Experimental factor	One in which the researcher has the responsibility for assigning the factor levels to the experimental units
Observational factor	One in which the researcher observes the level of the factor present on the experimental unit

Research projects may be described as one of two types:

Experimental study A research project that contains at least one experimental factor

Observational study A research project that contains only observational factors

One other distinction between types of studies can be made:

Prospective study A project in which the researcher chooses the experimental units, assigns levels of the experimental factors, notes levels of the observational factors, and measures the response variable at some future time

Retrospective study A project in which the response variable measurement already exists and the researcher is not trying to influence it. Instead, he or she is studying predetermined factors that may be related to the response variable measurements

Two types of retrospectives studies are

Case-control study One in which the researcher chooses a group of experimental units with a particular response variable measurement (usually presence of some disease state) and a control group with a different response variable measurement (usually absence of the disease state of interest) and compares these groups on their levels of a factor of interest

Cross-sectional survey One in which the factor levels and response variable measurements all are assessed at the same time

Parameter A single number used to describe a population of response variable measurements

Statistic A single number used to describe a P-sample of response variable measurements

2.13 FACTORS VERSUS RESPONSE VARIABLES

Some researchers find it difficult to determine which measurements are factors and which are response variables in a research project. It is important to understand this distinction, because the choice of statistical analysis depends on the number of factors being evaluated, the number of levels of each factor, and the type of response variable.

Remember that the factor (or independent variable) is that which, in the real world, can be administered or observed before the fact and the response variable (or dependent variable) is an outcome measure. Although factors and response variables are measured simultaneously in a cross-sectional survey study, the real-life distinction still exists. We generally wish to determine whether the set of response variable measurements obtained in a study is related to the factor level setting.

In a study, the factors and response variables are not necessarily set for the entire set of research hypotheses to be studied. Age, for example, may be a factor in one research hypothesis and a response variable in another research hypothesis.

You should realize that whether you are designing your own research project or evaluating someone else's project, you must be able to define and distinguish between the factors and response variables for each research hypothesis.

2.14 KEY POINTS

This chapter is the most important one in this book, as it defines the needed terminology for the design of and analysis of data in any research project. You must understand each of these terms before proceeding.

If you are not yet totally comfortable with all of these terms, proceed to Chapter 3, which presents numerous examples of research projects and defines the appropriate terms for each example. After you have read the examples in Chapter 3, each of the needed terms should be clear. If not, review the material in Chapters 2 and 3 until you have a thorough understanding of all terminology. The remaining chapters in this book should be much easier to read and understand if you have a good grasp of the material presented in this chapter.

REFERENCES

1. Colton, T. 1974. *Statistics in medicine*. Boston: Little, Brown.

2. Feinstein, A. R. 1977. *Clinical biostatistics*. St. Louis: Mosby. Chapters 2, 3, 12.

3. Feinstein, A. R. 1973. Clinical biostatistics XX: The epidemiologic trohoc, the ablatine risk ratio, and "retrospective" research. *Clin. pharmacol. Ther.* 14: 291.

4. Feinstein, A. R. 1970. Clinical biostatistics II: Statistics versus science in the design of experiments. *Clin. Pharmacol. Ther.* 11: 282.

5. Feinstein, A. R. 1970. Clinical biostatistics III: Components of the research objective. *Clin. Pharmacol. Ther.* 11: 432.

CHAPTER **3**

Examples Using the Needed Terminology

3.1 INTRODUCTION

A thorough understanding of the terminology in Chapter 2 is essential before you proceed through this book. To help you become familiar with the needed terminology, this chapter presents five examples, each with a detailed discussion of the research components introduced in Chapter 2. Even if you feel you clearly understand the terms in Chapter 2, read this chapter, as each of the examples will be discussed further in later chapters.

Project 3.1 A study of factors related to weight loss following gastric partition surgery

A researcher wishes to evaluate the initial weight loss of gastric partition surgery patients in the presence of various factors. Patients had been receiving a standard drug (Drug A) to help prevent diarrhea, a common malady after surgery. A new drug, Drug B, is now available. Drug B differs from Drug A in that it contains no atropine, which should produce less dryness in the mouth of a user. Thus, the researcher wishes to compare initial weight loss between people on each of these drugs.

Also, no program has been available to assist the patient with the choice of the necessary diet to follow after surgery. A new program is developed to assist each patient in determining his or her nutritional needs after surgery. The researcher wishes to compare initial weight loss in people not receiving this program with that of patients receiving this program. The researcher also wishes to determine whether initial weight loss is related to the length of hospitalization for the bypass surgery.

The objective of this project is **to study the relationship between antidiarrheic drug, nutrition plan, length of hospitalization and initial weight loss of patients having gastric partition surgery.**

The important terminology for this project is as follows:

Universe The group of all people who face gastric partition surgery. This surgery would be available to people who are at least 100 pounds over their ideal weight and had some health problem related to their weight, such as hypertension, diabetes, or musculoskeletal problems. Also, the surgery is advised only for people less than 50 years of age and who do not have peptic ulcers. People will be excluded from surgery if they have not explored all other alternatives or if they see this surgery as an "easy" solution to their problem. Also, people with psychological problems that might preclude their rehabilitation would be excluded from surgery.

Experimental unit An individual person from this universe

Response variable Initial weight loss achieved by a person undergoing this surgery (weight loss after one month, for example)

Population The collection of initial weight losses for each person undergoing this surgery

U-sample The collection of people participating in the study

P-sample The collection of initial weight losses for the people included in the study

Factors

QUALITATIVE FACTORS

Factor 1: Type of antidiarrheic drug
Level 1: Drug A
Level 2: Drug B

Factor 2: Nutrition program
Level 1: None
Level 2: New program

People having this surgery are placed on a drug and a particular nutrition program until they recuperate from the surgery. The goal is to compare these two drugs and two possible nutrition programs that the patients might receive to see whether these factors are related to weight loss. Because the levels of each factor simply categorize which type of drug and nutrition program a patient received, the factors are *qualitative*. Also, because a patient will be assigned to a level of each of these factors by the researcher, both of these factors are *experimental*.

QUANTITATIVE FACTOR

Factor 3: Length of hospitalization

The levels could be chosen in one of two ways. First, levels could be set at 7, 11, and 15 days, and patients could be assigned to be discharged at one of these times. Factor 3 would have three numerical levels in this situation. This factor also would then be *experimental*, because the researcher would be assigning each patient to one of these levels.

However, it may be difficult at the beginning of the research project to assign a date for discharge after surgery, because recovery will vary for different people, and a patient cannot be discharged until the doctors feel that the patient has recovered enough to leave the hospital. Therefore, no advance discharge date is assigned, and the researcher will simply record for each patient the length of stay in the hospital. In this situation, the factor is *observational*, because the researcher merely observes how long the patient remains in the hospital. The number of levels for this factor is the number of different days recorded for all experimental units. The number of levels in the observational factor certainly would be greater than the three levels for the factor if it were experimental.

One possible extraneous factor is initial weight. Another might be age, because younger people may shed pounds differently from the way older people do. Also, occupation might be an extraneous factor. People with outdoor or active jobs may be able to lose more pounds than do people with indoor desk jobs. Can you think of any other possible extraneous factors for this project? Extraneous factors are important to consider when you are choosing the experimental units to include in the study and when you are assigning factor levels to the experimental units. Chapters 8 and 11 will show how to control for extraneous factors at each of these stages of the research project.

This project is an example of a clinical trial study. Also, as it is presented, it is a prospective study. It also could be done as a retrospective study if patients have previously been exposed to both drugs and to the nutrition plan. Then these observational factors and weight loss could be obtained from the medical records.

Let us now look at another example where the experimental units are not living organisms.

Project 3.2 Estimating generic substitution in Florida

The state of Florida has a generic substitution law in which pharmacists may substitute generic drugs for name brand drugs if the drugs are chemically equivalent. The objective of this study is **to estimate the percentage of generically substituted prescriptions from all pharmacies in the state of Florida for a previous chosen month.**

The appropriate terms for this project are

Universe — All prescriptions that were filled by pharmacies in the state of Florida during the previous chosen month

Experimental unit — Each individual prescription in the universe

Response variable For each prescription, the verbal response *yes* or *no* would be recorded, where *yes* implies that a generic substitution was made and *no* implies that no substitution was made. (Note that a response variable does not have to be numerical, as shown by this example.)

Population The collection of all *yes* and *no* answers for all prescriptions in the state during the chosen month

U-sample The collection of prescriptions included in the study

P-sample The collection of *yes* and *no* answers for the prescriptions included in the study

Factor No factors are being studied in this project

The researcher, however, should consider possible extraneous factors that may influence the response variable. One possible extraneous factor might be geographic location. Pharmacies in a heavily urbanized area such as Miami may have a different attitude toward generic substitution from that in a more rural area such as the Florida panhandle. If this is the case, geographical location is an extraneous factor. Also, large-chain pharmacies may have a different attitude toward generic substitution from that of small-chain or independent pharmacies. If this is the case, type of pharmacy is an extraneous factor. Both these factors are qualitative, because their levels are categorical. Can you think of any other possible extraneous factors?

Most studies include at least one factor to evaluate, so this study is different in that regard. However, some studies are done in which there are no factors of interest. This study would be classified as a retrospective study, because the researcher will be going back through records and noting the response variable measurement (*yes* or *no*) from information contained in the record. This project is more practical as a retrospective study than as a prospective one. The researcher can get many more response variable measurements by leafing through records than by watching the pharmacist actually fill prescriptions and recording whether or not a substitution was made.

Project 3.3 Evaluation of the influence of SO_2 on breathing

A utility company is planning to burn a cheaper fuel that will release more sulfur dioxide (SO_2) into the air than does their current fuel. The Environmental Protection Agency will not approve the burning of this new fuel until the utility company proves that the SO_2 will not adversely influence people's breathing. The objective of this research project then is **to determine whether breathing of air plus SO_2 influences the breathing of either people with or people without breathing problems.**

Universe The collection of all people who are exposed to the air near the utility company. However, only healthy, nonsmoking

	adults will be studied. Also, asthmatics can have had no asthma attacks for the previous three months and must be taking no asthma medication.
Experimental unit	Each person included in this universe
Response variable	The response variable has not yet been chosen. It must be a measurement (or measurements) that accurately reflect how well a person is breathing. The next chapter deals with selecting the appropriate response variable in a research project. We shall return to this example at that time.
Population	The collection of the response variable measurements on each person in the universe
U-sample	The collection of people included in the study
P-sample	The collection of the response variable measurements on each person included in the study

Factors

QUALITATIVE FACTORS

Factor 1:	Group
Level 1:	Normals—no breathing problems
Level 2:	Asthmatics—people who have some sort of breathing problems
Factor 2:	Breathing what gas?
Level 1:	Air only
Level 2:	Air and SO_2

This study will evaluate the effect of breathing SO_2 on people without breathing problems and on people with breathing problems to determine whether SO_2 influences asthmatics more than it does people with no breathing problems. Also, a comparison will be made of people breathing air only with those breathing air and SO_2. Both factors are qualitative, because they categorize people into treatment groups. Also, Factor 1 is observational, because the researcher is merely observing into which group a person falls; and Factor 2 is experimental, because the researcher has control over which type of gas the participant is breathing.

QUANTITATIVE FACTOR

Factor 3:	Time breathing gas
Level 1:	Time 0 (baseline measurement)
Level 2:	Time .5 hour (h)
Level 3:	Time 1 h
Level 4:	Time 2 h
Level 5:	Time 3 h

People will be asked to sit in a chamber for three hours, and their breathing status will be measured at the above times. Because times are numerical measurements, Factor 3 is a quantitative factor; and in this case, the researcher can choose the settings for the levels. Therefore, the factor is also experimental: the researcher is assigning the levels to the participants. We shall discuss extraneous factors for this project in the next chapter, after we have chosen an appropriate response variable.

This project will most surely be a prospective study, because the response variable will be measured after the factor levels are assigned.

Project 3.4 Toothpaste comparison study

A manufacturing company wishes to compare a newly developed toothpaste to three existing commercial brands for flavor acceptance. People are selected to participate in this study and are assigned to use one of the four toothpaste brands for 90 days. At that time, their flavor acceptance will be measured and the toothpaste brands can be compared.

The objective of this project is **to determine whether a new toothpaste (Brand A) is at least equivalent to three other commercially available toothpastes (Brands B, C, and D) in flavor acceptance and gingivitis control.** For this project,

Universe All individuals between the ages of 6 and 65 who brush their teeth on a regular basis. People would be excluded from the study only if it was felt that they would not, or could not, complete the study or if they exhibited gross abnormalities in or around the oral cavity such as advanced periodontal conditions or excessive dental caries.

Experimental unit Each individual who satisfies the criteria in the above defined universe

Response variable A response from each person that will measure flavor acceptance. Let us ask a single question and record their flavor acceptance as:

1. Very pleasing taste
2. Somewhat pleasing taste
3. Taste is neither pleasing nor displeasing
4. Somewhat displeasing taste
5. Very displeasing taste

Gingivitis will be measured on the following scale by a dentist examining each patient:

1. No gingiva, no inflammation of gums
2. Gingivitis, some redness, slight inflammation of gums, no pain
3. Gingivitis, definite redness, frank inflammation, possible pain
4. Severe inflammation, angry red color, bleeding at slight touch

Population Collection of response variable measurements on each person in the universe

U-sample Collection of people included in the study

P-sample Collection of flavor acceptance measurements on people included in the study

QUALITATIVE FACTOR Type of toothpaste

Level 1: Brand A
Level 2: Brand B
Level 3: Brand C
Level 4: Brand D

This study could be done as either an experimental or an observational study. It would be experimental if the researcher could choose the people to participate in the study and assign to them the toothpaste they will use. If sex, age, and dental hygiene were identified as extraneous factors, the researcher could control for them by proper assignment of the toothpaste brands. Flavor acceptance then could be determined 90 days later.

The study would be observational if the researcher gathered the data by some sort of interview, such as by telephone or in a supermarket. In this type of study, the researcher would ask which type of toothpaste the respondent used and the flavor acceptance. Most likely, the respondent would respond favorably to the toothpaste flavor: otherwise, he or she would not be using it. Also, the researcher would not be able to control for the extraneous factors in this study. Finally, a grocery store interview would provide information only on people who *buy* the toothpaste and would provide nothing on other users. If telephone interviews were conducted during the day, the majority of respondents would be people not holding daytime jobs. Thus, you can see that for this particular project, an experimental study would be much more advantageous than an observational study.

If this study were experimental, it also would have to be prospective.

Project 3.5 A comparison of survival times in a cancer study

An oncologist would like to evaluate the survival rates of patients with oral cavity cancer who now face radiation therapy treatment. A standard dosing regimen has been used by this oncologist, and now a new dosing regimen has been proposed. Thus, the objective of this study is **to determine whether a new dosing regimen (Treatment A) is superior to a standard dosing regimen (Treatment B) in the survival time of patients with oral cavity cancer.** For this project,

Universe All patients with oral cavity cancer facing radiation therapy treatment. The only exclusion criterion would be distant metastasis or serious medical problem to prevent the use of this treatment.

Experimental unit	Each patient included in this universe
Response variable	Time of survival following surgery (in months)
Population	The collection of survival times for all patients in the universe
U-sample	The group of patients chosen to participate in this study
P-sample	The collection of survival times for patients participating in the study
QUALITATIVE FACTOR	Type of radiation therapy treatment
Level 1:	Treatment A
Level 2:	Treatment B

This study would be experimental and prospective, because the researcher would include patients who are ready to begin radiation therapy and would decide which treatment plan each patient would receive. Ethical considerations of patient assignment should be considered in this study. (This topic is discussed in Chapter 11.) Many extraneous factors may be present. Probably the most important extraneous factor influencing survival time is the stage at which the cancer is discovered. Age and general physical condition are two other factors that may influence a patient's survival time. Some researchers also may wish to include psychological outlook as another extraneous factor, because a patient with an optimistic outlook may survive longer than does a patient with a pessimistic outlook. Can you think of other possible extraneous factors?

3.2 RELATING THESE TERMS TO YOUR OWN RESEARCH PROJECT

By now, you should understand how to relate each of these terms to the objective of the research project. Referring to the objective of your project that you wrote down earlier, list your answers to these questions:

- What is the **universe of interest?**
- What is an **experimental unit?**
- What is (are) the **response variable(s)** to be measured? (You may not be able to answer this question yet.)
- What is (are) the **qualitative and quantitative factor(s)** to be studied?
- What are the **levels for each factor** listed above?
- Which of the above factors are **experimental,** and which are **observational?**
- Are there any **extraneous factors** that may affect the response variable measurements?
- Is this study **retrospective or prospective?**
- Is this study **experimental, case-control,** or a **cross-sectional survey?**

The next step in the experimental process is to decide on the most appropriate response variable, the one that will best achieve the objective of the project. Sometimes this procedure is straightforward, as in some of the examples in this chapter. In most projects, however, the researcher must choose the most appropriate response variable from a number of possibilities. The next chapter shows the different types of response variables that can be measured and how the researcher should choose the most appropriate one.

3.3 KEY POINTS

In Chapters 2 and 3, we have defined all the terminology you will need to proceed through this book and have provided examples to familiarize you with each of these terms. At this point, you may not realize why it is necessary to understand each of the defined terms, but each of them will be important in the chapters to follow on designing the research project. If you are still unclear on any of the terms, you should review them now so that they are clear to you as we move into the next chapters on research design.

CHAPTER 4

Step Two: Deciding What Type of Data to Collect

4.1 INTRODUCTION

After the objective of the research project has been clearly established, the researcher must decide how to achieve this objective. The next step in the research process will be to decide on an appropriate response variable. The researcher must consider two major criteria:

1. What is the most appropriate response variable that measures the phenomenon of interest and will allow me to achieve the research objective?
2. Which response variable can realistically be measured?

In some studies, the choice of response variable is clear-cut; but in many studies, the researcher must choose the most appropriate response variable from a number of possibilities. In many research projects, more than one response variable is measured. The researcher should be careful to choose the response variable (or set of response variables) that best satisfies the criteria mentioned.

There are four types of response variables: nominal, ordinal, discrete, and continuous. You must understand the differences among them and choose the one most appropriate for your particular project. In addition, the choice of statistical analysis depends on the type of response variable being analyzed.

Let us now look at each of these four types of response variable and see how to choose the most appropriate one for a research project.

4.2 EXAMPLE: TYPES OF RESPONSE VARIABLES

Let us evaluate the alternative types of response variables available in a research project.

Project 4.1 Employment status of people previously hospitalized for mental illness

A researcher is interested in studying people who have been hospitalized at least one time during their lives for mental illness. The objective of the project is **to determine whether the current employment status is different for the people who were hospitalized one time from what it is for people who were hospitalized more than one time.** In this project.

Universe — The group of all people who have been hospitalized for mental illness

Experimental unit — Each individual person hospitalized for mental illness

Factor — Number of times hospitalized for mental illness

This factor can be either qualitative or quantitative, depending on the levels that the researcher may choose. Let us look at examples of both types of factors.

Qualitative factor: — Hospitalization for mental illness

Level 1: — People who were admitted to the hospital only one time for mental illness

Level 2: — People admitted to the hospital more than one time for mental illness

Defining the levels this way would make the factor qualitative, because people are simply being categorized into one of two groups. The researcher might include in Level 1 only those people who have not been hospitalized for mental illness within the last five years. The researcher may feel that people who are readmitted for mental illness do so within a few years of their first admission and that if a patient is not readmitted within five years, he or she has made a successful adjustment. **To include people in Level 1 who have been hospitalized recently would cause problems, because it is yet unknown into which level these people eventually will be placed.** People thus could be misclassified, and erroneous conclusions about the universe of interest could result.

Quantitative factor: — Simply note the number of times that a person has been hospitalized for mental illness.

In either case, the hospitalization factor would be observational, because the researcher has no control over the number of hospitalizations.

This study is a cross-sectional survey if the data on hospitalization and employment status are obtained simultaneously. If the researcher decides to note the hospitalization status for each person selected for the study and to wait a few years to see into what type of employment the participant settles, the study is an observational, prospective study. This study could not be experimental, because the researcher has no control over assigning the factor levels. (See Chapter 2 if you need more information on prospective and retrospective studies.)

Let us now evaluate means of choosing an appropriate response variable. After the response variable is chosen, possible extraneous factors can be identified.

4.3 ALTERNATIVE TYPES OF RESPONSE VARIABLES FOR THIS EXAMPLE

Determining the response variable is the first step in achieving the research objective. The response variable must accurately measure the employment status of the people included in this study. The researcher might observe three possible response variables in these ways:

1. simply note for each person whether or not he or she was employed full-time;
2. record for each person whether he or she was unemployed, a manual laborer, a blue-collar worker, or a white-collar worker;
3. report each person's weekly income.

Each of these response variables yields different information about employment status. The researcher must decide which response variable, if any, most nearly achieves the objective of the research project. You will see later that there are problems with each of the above defined response variables. These are not the only response variables available. You may be able to think of more relevant ones.

In addition to choosing the most appropriate response variable, the researcher must consider whether it can be obtained practically. For example, data on these people might be available from the files of a local mental health clinic that has the responsibility of helping these people to return successfully to society after their hospitalization. The first two response variables that were suggested might be available in the patient's file, and hence are easily obtained. Salary data, however, may not be recorded in the files, and the researcher would have to contact each person to obtain this information. Problems such as out-of-date addresses, many long-distance telephone calls, confidentiality of data, and inability to find people at home might make these data too expensive and time consuming to collect. In that case, income data would not be collected even if they were deemed the most appropriate type.

4.4 TYPES OF RESPONSE VARIABLES

Response variables fit into four classifications. All response variables can be classified as **nominal, ordinal, discrete,** or **continuous.** The category into which your response variable falls determines the statistical analysis that will be chosen. Different statistical analyses exist for each type of response variable, and the appropriate analysis can be chosen only if the researcher knows the type of response variable that was measured. Let us look at the four different types.

4.4.1 Nominal Response Variables

The simplest form of response variable, the first type presented in Project 4.1, is **nominal.** Nominal data are verbal in nature. The response simply places an experimental unit in exactly one of a number of categories. In the previous example, the categories are *employed* and *unemployed.*

4.4.2 Ordinal Response Variables

The second type is **ordinal.** An ordinal response variable is similar to a nominal one in that it is verbal. (We shall show later that certain numerical response variables may also be considered to be on an ordinal scale.) With an ordinal response variable, however, the possible responses can be ranked in some manner. For example, *unemployed* pays less than does *manual* labor (only actual salary is included in the determination of income), which, in turn, generally pays less than does *blue-collar* labor; and finally, all these responses generally pay less than does *white-collar* labor. Thus, the ranking of the possible responses is

$$\text{unemployed} < \text{manual} < \text{blue-collar} < \text{white-collar}$$

and this ranking provides more information than does the simple knowledge of the category into which an experimental unit falls. Other examples of ordinal response variables would be *stage of breast cancer*, with levels A, B,C, and D; also

***COLIC*, WITH LEVELS**

none:	no crying that cannot be accounted for by the caregiver on some obvious basis
mild:	mild, brief episodes of unexplained crying or "fussiness" that are tolerable or easily controlled
moderate:	unexplained episodes of sustained crying, occurring often enough to be considered troublesome or distressing. Holding or rocking results in partial or inconsistent relief
moderately severe:	constant holding, rocking, or carrying baby is needed to prevent crying

severe: prolonged and intense episodes of crying or screaming, not lessened by any attempted method of control

***PLAQUE*, WITH LEVELS**

none: no detectable plaque on the tooth

slight: small amount of plaque, not extending more than 2 mm from the gingival margin

moderate: plaque covers up to half the exposed clinical crown of the tooth

severe: plaque covers more than half the exposed clinical crown

The possible outcomes for an ordinal response variable often require detailed explanations to allow for correct classification of an experimental unit. The categories must cover all possible occurrences without overlapping at all. There must be a clear and precise description of each possible outcome.

Often the categories of an ordinal response variable are classified numerically. For example, you may be asked to give an opinion on some issue by scoring the issue as follows:

1	strongly disagree
2	disagree
3	neutral
4	agree
5	strongly agree

The response measurements here are quantitative, yet the numbers really have no meaning. We cannot measure the difference between *strongly disagree* and *disagree* except to rank a 1 as a stronger feeling of disagreement than a 2. Therefore, the numerical scores could have been any numbers as long as the relative rankings were preserved. For example, the rankings

1	strongly disagree
3	disagree
8	neutral
9.5	agree
46	strongly agree

would be as valid as the integers 1 through 5 for this example, because

$$1 < 3 < 8 < 9.5 < 46$$

Therefore, although this response variable is numerical, it would be considered ordinal. The chosen statistical analysis would use only the *rankings* of the observations (i.e., 1, 2, 3, 4, 5) and not the actual measurements.

4.4.3 Discrete Response Variables

Both types of response variables presented so far, nominal and ordinal, refer to non-numerical or categorical measurements. The remaining two types of response variables discrete and continuous, refer to numerical or quantitative measurements. A **discrete** response variable can take on only certain numerical values, usually integers. If the experimental unit is a laboratory technician, a discrete response variable could be the number of errors made after the technician processes 100 laboratory tests. The response variable could be any integer from 0 to 100, but it would (we hope) take on only very small values. Other examples of discrete response variables would be the parity or number of children a woman has had, number of publications a university professor has, or the number of drugs a person may be taking at a given time. Each of these examples shows a response variable that can take on a countable number of numerical values.

4.4.4 Continuous Response Variables

The fourth type of response variable is continuous. A **continuous** response variable can take on any numerical value in a specified range. It is assumed that no two experimental units have exactly the same response variable measurements and that the accuracy of the measurements is limited by the person's or instrument's ability to obtain an exact measurement. Weight is an example of a continuous response variable. If the population of interest is all adults over the age of 18, the approximate range of weights is about 80 to 400 lb. However, a person does not necessarily weigh 150 lb, but may weigh 150.1 or 150.36 or 150.279 lb, or a weight that can be measured as exactly as possible by your scale. Thus, weight is said to be measured *on a continuum*, and no two people have *exactly* the same weight. Most physiological response variables, such as height, weight, blood pressure, heart rate, calcium, and potassium, are measured on continuous scales.

Continuous response variables can be divided into two categories, *interval* and *ratio*. However, both interval and ratio response variables usually are treated in the same way in data analysis, so we shall not go into the distinction between them.

For more information on these four types of response variables, or to read about the distinction between interval and ratio response variables, see references 1 through 3.

4.5 PARAMETERS AND STATISTICS FOR RESPONSE VARIABLES

The simplest nominal response variable is one with two categorical outcomes, such as *yes* or *no*, *dead* or *alive*, *normal* or *abnormal*. With this type of response, the researcher is interested in the percentage of successes that occur, such as the percentage of *yes* responses or the percentage of people alive or the percentage of abnormal test results. The parameter P denotes the percentage of successes that occur with any nominal response variable with two possible outcomes. If there are K categories of outcome, $K - 1$ parameters, denoted $P_1, P_2, \ldots, P_{K-1}$ would be defined to denote the percentage of response variable measurements occurring in those categories. (Note that P_K is not needed, because it will be known since the sum of P_1 to P_K will equal one.) We then can make inferences about these parameters using the statistics $\hat{P}_1$, $\hat{P}_2, \ldots$, which denote the percentage of successes in each category of outcome in the P-sample of response variable measurements.

If the response variable is ordinal, the appropriate population parameter is the *median*, denoted ε. The median is defined as the middle observation when all response variable measurements are ranked from low to high. If the number of observations is an even number, the median is the average of the two middle numbers. The statistic measuring the median of the P-sample is denoted as M.

Discrete and continuous response variables are numerical, and two parameters and statistics are associated with these types of response variables. The parameter μ denotes the average value of all numerical response variable measurements in the population; while σ^2, called the *variance*, measures the variability in the measurements. Most often, the inferences to be made are in terms of μ. The corresponding statistics representing the P-sample mean and variance are denoted $\bar{x}$ and s^2.

We shall discuss each of these parameters further in later chapters.

4.6 CHOOSING THE APPROPRIATE RESPONSE VARIABLE

The researcher must remember to decide on the response variable that 1) is most relevant to achieving the objective of the project and 2) realistically can be measured. If you are not careful, you may choose a response variable that cannot answer the research objective. For example, suppose that in Project 4.1 the researcher decides to measure a person's income from his or her job. Some people may have other income from welfare, a pension, insurance, or spouses who are employed. In this case, salary data alone for the experimental unit could be misleading. Also, unemployed people may only be collecting welfare or insurance, but the response variable as defined would be $0.00. In addition, some women may not have income-producing jobs if their spouses are employed and they have successfully performed the role of homemaker. It seems that they deserve more than a score of zero. Therefore, a more appropriate response variable might be total income for the family of an experimental unit, or something entirely different, if the dollar amounts obtained do not show the person's economic status and are not related to the employment status. You may feel that employment status is totally unrelated to economic status. Maybe some measurement of job satisfaction is more important than income as an indicator of employment status. This project points out the difficulty in defining an appropriate response variable in many studies. The important thing to remember is that choosing a relevant response variable to achieve an experimental objective is vital to the success of a research project and requires a great deal of thought.

If total family income is accepted as the most relevant response variable and you decide that it can be realistically measured, can you think of possible extraneous factors?

One might be the number of dependents in the family. A family with only two dependents can live more comfortably on $20,000 per year than can a family with six dependents. Therefore, number of dependents would be an extraneous factor. Amount of indebtedness might be another extraneous factor. A family owning a home and car outright can live comfortably on less money than can a family with a mortgage on the home and a loan on the car. A third possible extraneous factor would be age. A young person earning $15,000 may feel secure on the assumption that this income will rise with job advancement. A middle-aged or older person earning $15,000 may be very unhappy if this amount represents the peak of his or her earning potential.

In Chapter 2, we saw that the researcher must avoid having extraneous factors become confounded with factors of interest. In this study, the researcher must be confident that none of these possible extraneous factors interfere in this way.

4.7 EXAMPLES FOR DETERMINING RESPONSE VARIABLES

Let us now look at some other examples and follow the decision-making process that is used to determine the response variable for the research project.

Project 4.2 Evaluation of the influence of SO_2 on breathing

Refer to Project 3.3, where the objective of the experiment is **to determine whether the addition of SO_2 to the air influences breathing of people either with or without breathing problems.** The researcher must decide on an appropriate set of response variables (maybe only one) to achieve the objective of the project. These response variables must be selected so that they reflect a person's breathing ability.

This researcher chose these response variables:

Vital capacity A person takes a deep breath and holds it. He then blows out as much air as possible. Vital capacity is the amount of air blown out.

FEV_1 Forced expiratory volume measures how much air can be blown out in the first second of a breath.

MMFR Mid maximal expiratory flow rate measures the rate at which air is blown out at its peak.

FRC	Functional residual capacity measures the amount of air in the lungs at rest.
R_{aw}	The resistance of the airways measures the ease (or difficulty) with which air moves through the airways.

These response variables all are numerical measurements and would be considered continuous, because each can assume any value in a specified range. Each response variable also seems appropriate for determining how effectively a person is breathing and, hence, is adequate for answering the objective of the project.

Now that the appropriate response variables have been defined, let us try to identify some extraneous factors. One possible extraneous factor may be smoking habits. Nonsmokers may perform better on these breathing tests than do smokers. If so, smoking habits would be an extraneous factor. To control for this factor, only nonsmokers will be studied. Occupation may be another extraneous factor. People with outdoor or active jobs may be in better shape than are people with desk jobs, and hence they may perform better on the breathing tests. By the same reasoning, amount and type of exercise activity may be extraneous factors. Age, sex, and height all are potential extraneous factors. All these factors are qualitative except amount of exercise, which we might be able to quantify (i.e., hours of exercise per day).

Project 4.3 Evaluation of educational procedures to reduce prejudice of grade school children

The objective of this researcher's project is **to determine whether a newly developed educational procedure can improve the attitude of grade school children in their prejudice toward the handicapped.** The appropriate terms for this project are

Universe	All grade school children
Experimental unit	Each individual grade school child
Qualitative factor	Type of education received
Level 1:	No education
Level 2:	Newly developed educational procedure

This factor is experimental, because the children will be assigned by the researcher to one of the two levels. This study is prospective, because the response variable measurements will be obtained from the experimental units at a future time after they are assigned to factor levels. In this particular project, response variable measurements also will be taken before assignment of factor levels, and these measurements will be referred to as **baseline values.** These baseline values will enable the researcher to identify a child's prejudice at the beginning of the study and then measure the change in prejudice after the educational program ends. One group of children will receive the new educational procedure. The other group will receive no education and thus will serve as a control. A control group is included because the attitude of the children may be affected mainly by the presence of the researcher in the classroom, rather than by a learning effect. This phenomenon is known as the Hawthorne effect; it will be discussed in more detail in Chapter 11. We can measure this effect by studying the control group and then making a comparison between the response variable before and after treatment.

We now must select an appropriate response variable so that we can evaluate the research objective. The response variable must be able to identify children who are prejudiced against the physically handicapped and also should measure the degree of prejudice.

A grade school class of 30 nonhandicapped children and four handicapped children has been selected to provide the children for this project.

One possible response variable would be simply to ask the nonhandicapped students whether or not they are prejudiced against the handicapped and to record a *yes* or *no* response for each student. The response variable then would be nominal. This approach probably is not satisfactory, however, because the students may not answer truthfully for fear of admitting their prejudice. Therefore, another more appropriate response variable should be selected.

Consider a piece of paper containing the names of all class members. Each person in the class is given a copy of the sheet and instructed to score each classmate as follows:

1 if he or she considers the classmate a friend,

2 if he or she is neutral to the classmate,

3 if he or she dislikes the classmate.

Then, on each paper, the points given to the four handicapped students are totaled, and each nonhandicapped student in the class has a score measuring his or her prejudice. The range of scores will be from four to 12, where a four indicates no prejudice because each handicapped student was scored a 1, and 12 indicates much prejudice because each handicapped student was scored a 3. Then we might choose all students scoring over six as being prejudiced or we might use their determined numerical score.

A problem arises with this scoring scheme in that it is possible to misclassify a student. For example, a student getting a score of 12 would be considered prejudiced; yet this student may have scored *every* member of the class as a 3. This student is not necessarily prejudiced against the handicapped, but instead dislikes the entire class. It seems that we should take into account the scoring of the nonhandicapped students also. Here are two possible classification schemes.

1. Each nonhandicapped student in the class scores the remaining 29 nonhandicapped students and 4 handicapped students. The average of the 29 nonhandicapped scores and the average of the four handicapped students are computed. A student is said to be prejudiced if the nonhandicapped average is less than 2 and the handicapped average is more than 2.
2. Compute the scores as above and, for each nonhandicapped student, compare the scores they assigned to the handicapped and nonhandicapped

students. Use an appropriate statistical test of the hypothesis that the distribution of scores for the nonhandicapped students is similar to the scores for the handicapped students. (Note: Do not be concerned about the details of such a test at this point.) If the statistical test rejects this hypothesis and the handicapped scores are significantly higher than are the nonhandicapped scores, then the student would be said to be prejudiced.

Both methods have drawbacks. The first method is subjective, in that 2 has no real meaning as a cutoff point other than that it represents the "average" response. The second method may not yield statistical significance even if the child is prejudiced because of the small number of handicapped children being ranked. A numerical response variable would be to use the difference between the average scores for the non-handicapped and handicapped students. This example shows the difficulty in choosing an appropriate response variable. It may not be possible to select a completely accurate and objective response variable for this research project.

If we can determine an appropriate response variable measuring prejudice, then we should consider possible extraneous factors. In this project, possible extraneous factors may include sex, race, intelligence quotient (IQ), parents' socioeconomic status, and parents' education. If we are concerned about the effect of any of these extraneous factors on the response variable and the comparison of the two factor levels, we must control for them. Methods for accomplishing this control will be discussed in Chapter 11.

4.8 MEASUREMENT ERRORS IN THE RESPONSE VARIABLE

To achieve the research objective, we must choose the most appropriate response variable that adequately measures the phenomenon of interest. We also must be concerned that the response variable is being measured accurately and precisely.

One common form of measurement error is machine error. For example, if a blood pressure cuff shows a reading of 140/80, do those readings accurately reflect the blood pressure for that person, or could there be error? If error is suspected in the machine-recorded response variable measurements, then this error should be quantified by repeated measures on the same person under similar conditions to determine how precise these measures are. In data analysis, the objective will be to determine and measure all sources that contribute to the variation in the response variable measurements.

Other considerations dealing with measurement error are validity, reliability, sensitivity, and specificity.

4.8.1 Validity and Reliability of a Response Variable

Project 4.3 is a good example of the difficulty often experienced in the choice of a suitable response variable. This choice becomes especially difficult when one is measuring a subjective phenomenon such as prejudice, depression, employment status, severity of disease, or pain relief. For many subjective measurements, there is no single straightforward measurement, and the researcher usually has to develop his or her own instrument. In these situations, one should be concerned with the validity and reliability of the instrument. The **validity** of an instrument is its ability to measure accurately the phenomenon of interest, while the **reliability** measures the ability of the instrument consistently to produce accurate measurements when used by other researchers or by the same researcher on the same experimental units repeatedly. There are many types of validity and reliability, such as content validity, criterion-related validity, construct validity, and predictive validity. Reliability can be evaluated by its stability, internal consistency, and equivalence. We shall not discuss these concepts further here, but reference 4 gives more details.

4.8.2 Sensitivity and Specificity of a Response Variable

A diagnostic test generally is used to determine the presence or absence of a disease. The response variable in this situation is on a nominal scale, because it is a *yes* or *no* outcome. The researcher must be concerned with a correct diagnosis for the test. The **sensitivity** of a test measures its ability to confirm correctly the presence of the disease (or avoid a false negative), while the **specificity** is the test's ability to diagnose correctly the absence of the disease (or avoid a false positive). Obviously, a diagnostic test whose sensitivity and specificity are not very good will produce unreliable response variable measurements, and no valid conclusions can be drawn from the study. Thus, the researcher should determine the specificity and sensitivity of a diagnostic test he is using. More information on the sensitivity and specificity of a diagnostic test can be found in references 3 and 5 through 7.

4.9 DETERMINING THE CATEGORY OF YOUR RESPONSE VARIABLE

For the prejudice example in Project 4.3, the response variables might be considered ordinal, discrete, or continuous. Although the measurements being made are numerical, some researchers may believe that the measurements are more accurately described as ordinal. If that is the case, the response variable should be considered ordinal. The point is that not all researchers would agree on the classification of the response variable.

Another response variable that often is misclassified is time to some occurrence. This error is easily made if not all experimental units have experienced the occurrence by the end of the study. Consider Project 3.5, in which the response variable was time of survival in months following surgery for stage II oral cavity cancer. The time to an occurrence in this project is time to death. This response variable might be considered on a continuous scale because the response is numerical, and no two patients would have exactly the same length of survival. Suppose this study included 10 patients and they were followed for five years. The survival time of each patient is given below. Eight of the 10 patients have died from this cancer, including patient H, who died at the end of the study. Patients I and J are still alive. What numerical response should be assigned to them? In some studies of this type, I have seen scores of 60 assigned to patients I and J. This assignment provides false information, as patients I and J are considered to have died at the end of the study, similarly to patient H. It would be more appropriate to consider the response variable to be on an ordinal scale and to assign patients I and J a score of 61 or higher. As pointed out earlier, for an ordinal response variable, the ranks of the measurements are used instead of the actual measurements. Therefore, a 61 (or higher number) would signify that patients I and J lived longer than did patient H, but would not measure how much longer if treated as ordinal.

Table 4.1 Survival times after surgery for oral cavity cancer

Patient	*Survival time (months)*
A	3
B	8
C	11
D	12
E	22
F	38
G	42
H	60
I	alive
J	alive

In the analysis of *this particular project*, the survival times usually are grouped into six- or 12-month clusters. This procedure certainly would put the clustered responses on an ordinal scale. *In general*, however, a numerical response variable, whether treated as numerical or as ordinal, should not have the responses grouped into clusters. For example, the response variable age is continuous, yet it may be considered ordinal in some studies for analysis purposes. We often see age presented by various categories, one common categorization being $1 = <10$, $2 = 10–19$, $3 = 20–29$, $4 = 30–39$, $5 = 40–49$, $6 = 50–59$, $7 = 60+$. This approach certainly puts the response on an ordinal scale, but it reduces available information and actually provides erroneous information. For example, two people aged 10 and 19 both are classified as 2, and thus valuable information regarding the difference in their ages is lost. Yet two people aged 19 and 20 are classified differently, one as a 2 and the other as a 3. This information is really erroneous, as these two people actually are similar in age. Also, a different classification, such as <15, 15–24, 25–34, 35–44, 45–54, 55–64, and 65+ or one using five-year intervals, could yield different sets of measurements, and the results of the statistical analysis could change depending on which categorization was used. All these problems can be avoided if we use each person's actual age instead of grouping them into intervals.

4.10 HOW RESPONSE VARIABLE TYPE INFLUENCES THE CHOICE OF STATISTICAL ANALYSIS

As we have been showing throughout this chapter, after the response variable has been chosen, its type must be considered. Should the response variable be considered as nominal, ordinal, discrete, or continuous? This choice is not always easy; but we must make this decision, because the choice of statistical analysis depends on the type of response variable measured. Different analyses exist for nominal, ordinal, and numerical response variables. Because the choice of type of response variable is not automatic, different researchers may not agree on the type, and hence they also would not agree on the choice of statistical analysis. If you are presenting the statistical results of your work at a national meeting, in a scientific journal, to a thesis committee, or to a grant review team, someone may ask why you did a t test instead of a chi-square test, or why you did a one-way analysis of variance (ANOVA) instead of a Kruskal-Wallis one-way ANOVA. Your answer should not be "This is the test my statistician suggested" or "I only learned a t test in my one statistics course" or "This is the only test programmed into my calculator." Your choice of statistical test should be based on your research design and the type of response variable measured.

Remember that you, the researcher, must accept complete responsibility for your research work and the results that are obtained. Thus, you should understand the decision-making process that goes into choosing the statistical analysis and interpreting the results. This part of your research should not be accepted blindly, even if it is carried out by an experienced statistician, because *you* are the one who must justify the results to your peers, and hence, you must be able to answer questions about the choice of analysis and its interpretation.

4.11 CAN YOU AFFORD TO MEASURE THE RESPONSE VARIABLE?

After determining some appropriate response variables for the research project, you must consider whether the resources (usually time and money) are available to collect this type of response variable. **A common mistake made by first-time**

researchers is to overestimate the amount of data that can be collected or the ease with which it can be collected. Collect a small sample of data, if you can, before finalizing the choice of response variable to be sure that the selection of the response variable is *practical* as well as *relevant*.

Let us take a look at two examples that illustrate this idea.

Project 4.4 Estimating generic substitution in Florida

Refer to Project 3.2, which had the objective of **estimating the percentage of generically substituted prescriptions from all pharmacies in the state of Florida for a particular month.**

The researcher planned to hire pharmacy graduate students to go into the selected pharmacies and collect the response variable measurements. A student would work all day in one pharmacy, reviewing as many prescriptions as possible. The researcher felt that a person could review about 1000 prescriptions in an eight-hour day and thus requested funding for 60 workdays to collect an adequate amount of data. After carefully designing a valid project and looking after all details, the researcher was funded and prepared to begin the data collection stage of the research project. At this time, the researcher went to a local pharmacy to collect some response variable measurements and then found out that only about 500 prescriptions could be studied in a workday. Thus only 50 percent of the desired measurements could be collected, and some of the researcher's objectives had to be altered. The researcher should have taken the sample earlier, and the design of the project and request for funding could have been altered to suit the situation better.

Project 4.5 Evaluation of a new drug to test epilepsy

Drug X has just been developed to treat epilepsy. A graduate student in pharmacy wishes to compare Drug X to a standard drug, Drug Y, which is used currently to treat epileptics at a local institution for mentally retarded people. The objective of this study is **to evaluate the relationship between type of drug administered (Drug X and Drug Y) and the epileptic seizure rate of mentally retarded people.**

A group of these people will be selected from a nearby institution for the mentally retarded, and each person in the study will be an experimental unit. The only qualitative factor in this project is drug type, and the two levels are 1) Drug X and 2) current drug used. This factor is experimental, because the researcher will assign the people to receive a particular drug. Also, the study is prospective, because the response variable will be obtained at a time after the people are assigned to the drugs. The researcher decides that an appropriate response variable will be monthly epilepsy rate. Since each person will experience a few seizures per month, the researcher decides to follow each person for at least three months to get an accurate measure of his or her seizure rate for the current drug used. The researcher then discovers that only 12 people are available for the study at the local institution. The information on occurrence of an epileptic attack would be provided by the house parent of each person in the study. To be confident that all the measurements are accurate, the researcher would have to check with each house parent daily to find out whether the participant suffered a seizure. The researcher would do so for three months to determine the seizure rate for each participant on his or her current drug and then repeat it for three months while the participants received Drug X. Therefore, this project entails checking with about 12 house parents daily for six months and also making sure that the participants take their new drug for the last few months of the study. After all this time and effort, the researcher will be rewarded with a total of 24 measurements, the seizure rate for each participant before and after he or she receives Drug X. Even if the monthly seizure rates are not averaged for each person, there will be 72 observations, but all from only 12 people. The amount of information obtained is not very great. Is it worth doing all this work for the limited information that can be obtained? If this information is impractical to obtain, the researcher must choose another response variable that is more practical, choose another setting for the study, or give up on this project entirely.

4.12 CHOOSING THE MOST APPROPRIATE RESPONSE VARIABLE

In any research project, four different types of response variables can be collected, and you must try to choose the most relevant and appropriate response variable that will help to achieve the objective of your research project. For the project whose objective you listed in Chapter 2, try to list different types of response variables that might be appropriate. Which of the response variables is most relevant for your research project? Is it practical to measure the chosen response variable? The questions that a response variable should answer positively are

- What are some appropriate response variables for this project?
- Which of these response variables allow me to achieve the objective of my project?
- Which of these response variables most objectively measure the phenomenon that I wish to study?

  Which of these response variables can I realistically expect to collect with the resources available to me?
- For each response variable to be measured, what is its type—nominal, ordinal, discrete, or continuous?

4.13 KEY POINTS

You must consider a number of important points in your research project. First, be sure to choose response variables that are relevant to your research objective and practical to obtain. If you are planning your research project for a thesis, dissertation, or a granting agency, there is a good chance that you will be quizzed as to the appropriateness of the chosen response variables and the practicality of obtaining those measurements.

You probably also will be questioned as to the statistical analysis you plan to use to analyze the data and answer the research objective. Thus, it is important to determine the type of each response variable—nominal, ordinal, discrete, or continuous—as this step is necessary as one justification of the chosen statistical analysis. Remember that, for analysis purposes, a response variable may be treated on a lower level. Usually, in this case, a numerical response variable is treated as ordinal.

4.14 THE NEXT STEP

Now that all the factors and response variables have been defined, you should lay out a data collection sheet that will contain all data for a single experimental unit. It is especially advantageous to design the data collection sheet now if your project is being described in a grant proposal. Too often researchers make only general statements in their grant proposals as to the data they will collect. If the researcher is not very specific on this point, the grant review team cannot review the grant adequately, and your proposal will receive a negative review because of lack of clarity.

Including the actual data collection form provides specific information and allows the grant review team to become much more familiar with your proposed data. The data can still be changed and the data collection sheet reorganized, and in fact, the grant review team probably will make suggestions to improve it. But by including an initial version of your data collection form, you will show that you have given much thought to the data you will collect and that you are ready to begin data collection.

REFERENCES

1. Siegel, S. 1956. *Nonparametric statistics for the behavioral sciences.* New York: McGraw-Hill. Pp. 21–30.

2. Agresti, A., and Agresti, B. F. 1979. *Statistical methods for the social sciences.* San Francisco: Dellen Publishing Co. Pp. 15–17.

3. Colton, T. 1974. *Statistics in medicine.* Boston: Little, Brown & Co. Pp. 90–92.

4. Polit, D., and Hungler, B. 1978. *Nursing research: Principles and methods.* Philadelphia: J. B. Lippincott Co.

5. Rimm, A. A., Hartz, A. J., Kalbfleisch, J. H., Anderson, A. J., and Hoffmann, R. G. 1980. *Basic biostatistics in medicine and epidemiology*. New York: Appleton-Century-Crofts. Pp. 56–58.

6. Feinstein, A. R. 1977. *Clinical biostatistics*. 1977. St. Louis: C. V. Mosby. Pp. 214–226.

7. Feinstein, A. R. 1975. Clinical biostatistics XXXI: On the sensitivity, specificity, and discrimination of diagnostic tests, *Clin. Pharmacol Ther*. 17: 104–116.

CHAPTER 5

Step Three: Designing a Data Collection Form

5.1 INTRODUCTION

Now that you have identified all the data to be collected, you should lay out your data collection sheet. If you will be recording all the data yourself, you may not think of designing a data collection form but simply plan on methodically reporting all the data on one large sheet of paper, if the project is a small laboratory study. However, at some point the data must be put into a form that can be read by a computer. Data must be laid out appropriately for data processing. A data collection sheet filled out initially allows you to avoid transcribing the data later. Thus, you save time and eliminate transcription errors.

If you are collecting data on a questionnaire that will be filled out by many people, the form of the questionnaire (your data collection form) becomes very important. Questions must be stated clearly so that the reader will understand them, appropriate responses must be given, and answer spaces must be provided and clearly labeled so that you can easily determine the respondent's answer to a question.

Data processing usually is done manually. You should design the data collection form so that it is clear and convenient for the person filling out the form, and also for the person processing the data.

The most common methods of processing data are card keypunching, terminal entry, optical scanning, and paper tape. We shall discuss only the keypunching of computer cards here, but this discussion would apply to any form of manual data processing.

Let us now consider the points necessary in the design of an efficient data collection form.

5.2 GENERAL DESIGN CONSIDERATIONS

A data collection form should be designed for any research project in which the data will be analyzed on a computer. The data must be processed to be read by the computer. We shall assume that the form of processing will be card keypunching.

The data collection form should be designed with the following purposes in mind: 1) to provide an efficient, easy-to-use instrument for the person(s) recording the data and 2) to provide the data processor (keypuncher) with a form that can be clearly read, interpreted, and followed. The computer card onto which the data is keypunched is simply a card (usually manila colored) about the size of a dollar bill, containing 80 columns in which numbers, letters, or special symbols can be punched. An example of a punched computer card is shown in Figure 5.1.

Data for each experimental unit in the study will be punched onto a separate computer card. If more information is collected than can fit onto one card, or if information is collected at more than one time for each experimental unit, then multiple cards would be used to provide the complete information obtained from an experimental unit.

The information to be recorded on the computer card for an experimental unit falls into these categories:

Demographic information will uniquely identify the experimental unit and provide basic descriptive information, such as name, identification number (i.e., social security number or hospital number), sex, race, income level, occupation, etc.

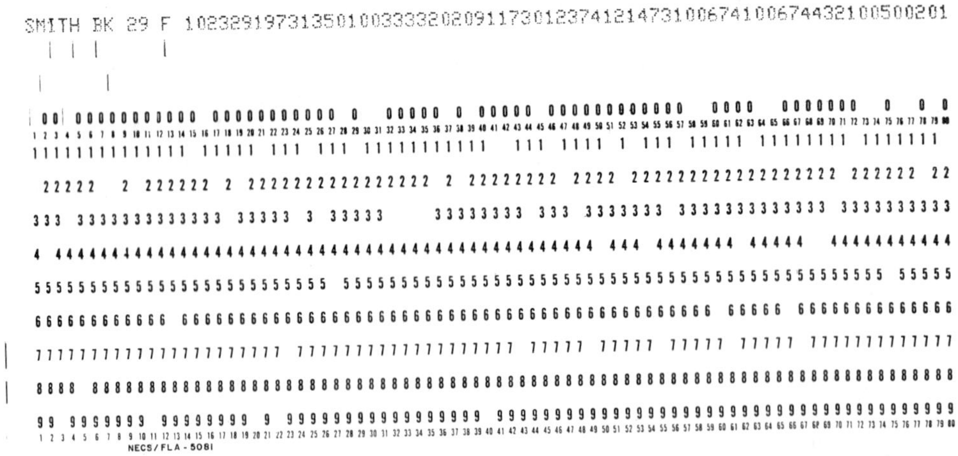

SMITH BK 29 F 10232919731350100333320209117301237412147310067410067443210050020l

NECS/FLA-5081

Figure 5.1 Computer card.

Extraneous factor levels will be noted for each potential extraneous factor that was identified. (Note that the extraneous factors may overlap some of the demographic measurements.)

Factor levels for all factors of interest in the research project

Response variable measurements for each response variable being studied

Let us now look at how to code this information for efficient data processing and data management.

5.3 CODING THE RESEARCH DATA

The first decision is to choose the demographic information to include on the data collection form. If you are unsure whether a certain measurement is important, you should include that information on the data collection form. Collecting measurements that may never be used in the analysis is less of a problem than is needing some measurement later that was not included on the data collection form.

One demographic measurement that should be included on virtually all data collection forms is a unique identifying name or number (ID) for each experimental unit in the study. If you have this ID, you always can go back from the computer card to the data collection form to verify measurements that look suspicious. The ID also enables you to link data on several computer cards together. A computer program could be written to link the measurements together, as long as a unique ID for each experimental unit is recorded on each of its computer cards. Commonly used IDs are social security numbers or hospital numbers. Names of people and birth dates can be used for identification, but they are not necessarily unique.

Even if the experimental units are not originally numbered in some way, such as with animals or questionnaires, a unique ID should be assigned, such as 001 through 100 if 100 animals are used in a study.

Next, you must decide which other demographic measurements may be of interest and should be included. Some measurements also may turn out to be the potential extraneous factors in the research project. Frequently reported demographic measurements include sex, race, age, income level, occupation, and marital status. These demographic measurements, as well as ID, all can be coded in one of two ways on the data collection form. Measurements such as age, height, and weight are numerical and are coded as such. Other demographic measurements, such as sex and race, are not numerical. These nonnumerical demographic measurements can be coded as either numeric or alphameric. Sex could be coded either as M and F or as 1 and 2, where 1 would refer to one sex and 2 to the other. Many people prefer to code all measurements numerically for data processing and data management. A numeric coding scheme could cause problems, however, if more than one person is recording measurements or if one person is recording measurements at different times.

All recorders would have to remember which sex is coded as 1 and which as 2 and remain consistent throughout the data coding process. Most computer programs can read alphameric codes as easily as numeric ones. Thus, you should use alphameric codes for non-numerical measurements if there is any chance of confusion.

In either coding situation, you next must decide how many columns to allocate for each demographic response.

After the demographic responses all have been coded and allocated to columns on the computer card, you then must follow the same process for the extraneous factors, the factor levels, and the response variable measurements.

If the data require multiple cards, then a column on the card is used to denote card number. Column 80 generally is used for this purpose. Thus, if five computer cards are required to contain all the data for an experimental unit, the identification number should be repeated on each card, and the cards should be numbered from one to five in column 80.

Let us now look at some examples of data collection forms that demonstrate these principles.

5.4 EXAMPLES OF DATA COLLECTION FORMS

Project 5.1 Drug utilization at a center for mentally retarded

A pharmacy researcher wishes to evaluate the drug use of a group of mentally retarded people at a particular government-sponsored center. It is of prime importance **to compare drug usage rates for people at this center before and after implementation of a new drug-distribution method.** The important terms to define for this project are as follows:

Universe	all mentally retarded people at similar government centers
Experimental unit	each person at one of these centers
Response variable	number of drugs taken by a person
Observational qualitative factor	drug distribution method
Level 1:	old method
Level 2:	new method

This study is a cross-sectional survey, because the data will be gathered from the records at the center. This information already exists, and no future data will be collected. In addition to the response variable defined above, the researcher is interested in obtaining more drug information on each person. Thus, for each experimental unit, the researcher wishes to know each drug taken, the dosage and number of times taken daily for each drug, in what form it is taken, which doctor prescribed it, and whether it is treating an acute or a chronic condition. The researcher decides that six is the maximum number of drugs that any person is taking, so the data collection form must be designed to collect this information on six drugs. Let us now look at one means of setting up this data collection form.

The first step will be to establish an ID to identify uniquely each experimental unit. The researcher will use the first four columns of the computer card for the first four letters of the person's last name and the fifth column for the first initial. This method will quickly identify people who may be selected out of the total group at the center. The main ID will be the person's six-digit ID number, which is a unique number assigned to each person when he or she first comes to the center. This number will appear in columns 6 through 11 of the computer card. This information may be laid out as in Figure 5.2.

The remaining demographic information to be obtained will be IQ, sex, race, age, and weight. A single column will be used to identify the IQ level of a person. Column 12 will contain one of the following codes:

Code	*IQ*
1	0–24
2	25–39
3	40–54
4	55–69
5	70–84
6	85+

Sex will be coded in column 13 as

M male
F female

and race will be coded in column 14 as

W white
B black
O other

Age in years is a two-digit number and will be coded in columns 15 and 16. Weight in pounds is a three-digit number and will be coded in columns 17

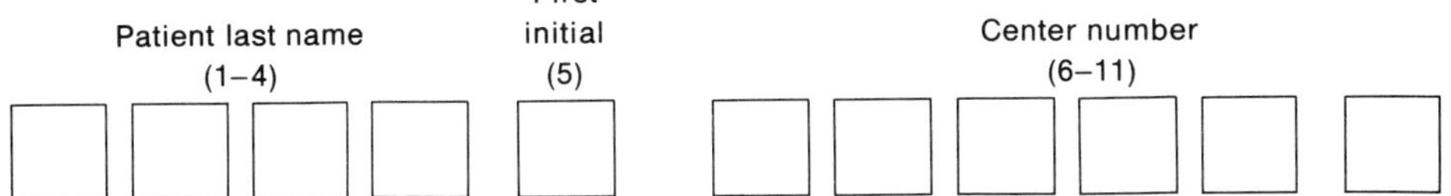

Figure 5.2 The first 11 columns of a computer-card data collection form for Project 5.1.

through 19. Note that age is specified in years and weight in pounds as the units of measurement. This restriction prevents, for example, a situation in which one person codes weight in pounds and another in kilograms. The data collection form should be coded as specifically as possible.

Column 20 will denote the drug distribution method that was in use at the time when these drugs were dispensed. A 1 will denote the old method and a 2, the new method. These measurements may be laid out as in Figure 5.3.

Next, we need to obtain information on each drug taken by each person. Each drug will be identified by a unique five-digit numerical drug code that we design. The code is designed to allow drugs to be combined in various ways, such as by similar drug classes. We also must identify the dosing interval (DI) for each drug. We shall need a single digit to code the following possible doses. Note that all drug dosages have been converted to a common unit-dose scale.

Codes for drug doses

Code	*Unit Doses*	*Times Administered Daily*
1	1	1
2	1	2
3	1	3
4	1	4
5	2	1
6	2	2
7	2	3
8	2	4
9	>8	

We shall need a single column to code the route of administration as follows:

1 oral
2 intravenous
3 rectal
4 intramuscular
5 subcutaneous
6 topical
7 nasal

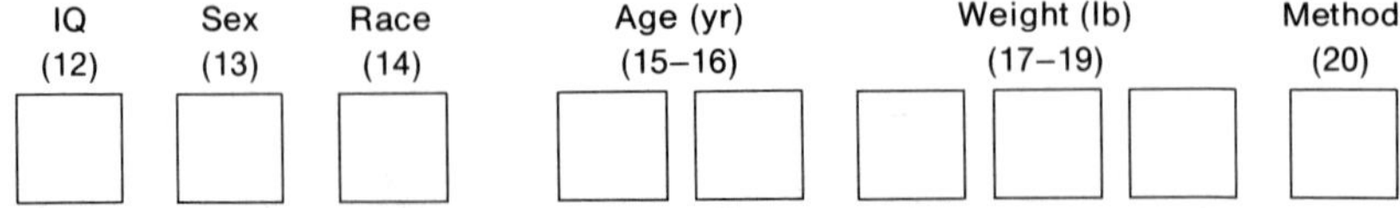

Figure 5.3 Coding further information for Project 5.1.

8	otic
9	ophthalmic

A two-digit code will identify the doctor who prescribed the drug, because about 50 doctors can prescribe them. Finally, a single letter will denote whether the drug is being used to treat an acute or a chronic condition. The possible codes will be

A	acute condition
C	chronic condition
N	not determined

Thus, for each drug we need 10 columns to gather the desired information. For the first drug, the data might be laid out as in Figure 5.4.

Because there are six possible drugs for each person, we shall need a total of 60 columns to code all the drug information. Because 20 columns on the computer card were used to code the demographic information and the single factor of interest, the additional 60 columns for drug information fill the 80-column field on the computer card. Note that the response variable of interest is the number of drugs being taken by a person, and this datum is not coded anywhere on the data collection form. A computer program can be written to tabulate the number of drugs being taken from the information on the computer card. If a person is taking fewer than six drugs, the appropriate columns simply would be left blank.

The complete data collection form now is shown in Figure 5.5. Note the flow of responses from left to right in even rows, which simplifies the reading of the form by the keypuncher. Also, the blocks are large so that the numbers and letters can be entered legibly. Remember that it takes time and money to have the data keypunched. The easier the forms are to read, the faster the data can be entered. Also, the number of errors in keypunching can be kept to a minimum.

To eliminate errors in keypunching, have the punched data verified for accuracy. Professional keypunchers have a machine to facilitate this procedure. If you do your own keypunching, verifying the data can be a tedious and boring job, but *do not underestimate the importance of verifying data*. It is poor practice to be careful in collecting the proper data and then not to check to

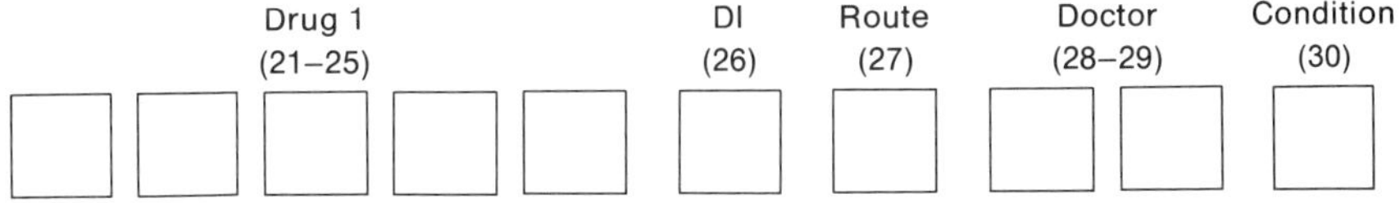

Figure 5.4 Drug information for Project 5.1.

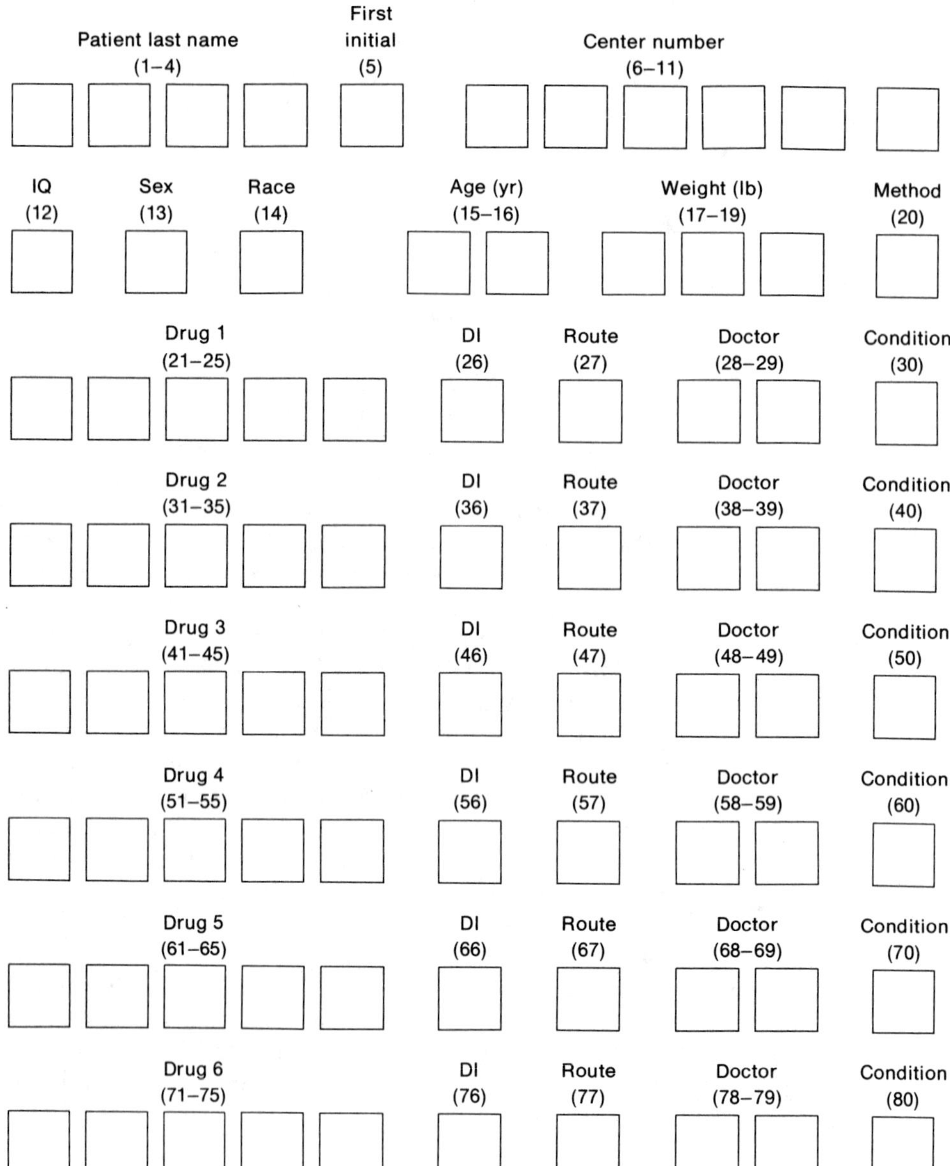

DRUG UTILIZATION REVIEW PROGRAM

Patient last name (1–4) | First initial (5) | Center number (6–11)

IQ (12) | Sex (13) | Race (14) | Age (yr) (15–16) | Weight (lb) (17–19) | Method (20)

Drug 1 (21–25) | DI (26) | Route (27) | Doctor (28–29) | Condition (30)

Drug 2 (31–35) | DI (36) | Route (37) | Doctor (38–39) | Condition (40)

Drug 3 (41–45) | DI (46) | Route (47) | Doctor (48–49) | Condition (50)

Drug 4 (51–55) | DI (56) | Route (57) | Doctor (58–59) | Condition (60)

Drug 5 (61–65) | DI (66) | Route (67) | Doctor (68–69) | Condition (70)

Drug 6 (71–75) | DI (76) | Route (77) | Doctor (78–79) | Condition (80)

Figure 5.5 Data collection form for Project 5.1.

make sure that the correct responses have been keypunched. Ignoring the verification process is false economy and can easily lead one to draw incorrect conclusions.

Project 5.2 Data collection form for gastric partition study

The form used in this research project is reprinted with the permission of Margaret C. Duerson, Department of Surgery, J. Hillis Miller Health Center, University of Florida. Refer to Project 3.1, which had as its main objective **to study the relationship between type of antidiarrheic drug, nutrition plan, length of hospitalization, and the initial weight loss of patients undergoing gastric partition surgery.**

A lot of information is collected on people entering the hospital for this surgery before they undergo it. Demographic information includes past medical history, current physical status, and many laboratory test results. Other measurements are collected just before and soon after surgery. Finally, various measurements are collected each time a patient returns for a follow-up visit. Thus, this project involves the collection of a large amount of data measured over a long period of time. Also, the number of follow-up visits and length of time between visits differs for each person involved in the study. The result is a much more complex collection scheme than that in Project 5.1.

In Figure 5.6, you can see part of the data collection form that is used in this research project. Each card begins with the nine-digit identification number (social security number in this project), and each card ends with the card number in the last two columns. The first five cards contain a patient's baseline physiological and demographic information.

The first card contains very basic registration information, such as sex, marital status, date of birth, name, address, and occupation. Sex is coded as F or M and marital status is coded as

1 single
2 married
3 separated
4 divorced

Name, address, and occupation all are spelled out.

The second card then covers the patient's physical history. The codes for the non-numerical data are shown in Table 5.1. Columns 35 through 54 are for the coded illnesses. For each person, each illness is coded into one of the pairs of columns. It is assumed that none have had more than 10 of the listed illnesses, because that is the maximum number that can be reported.

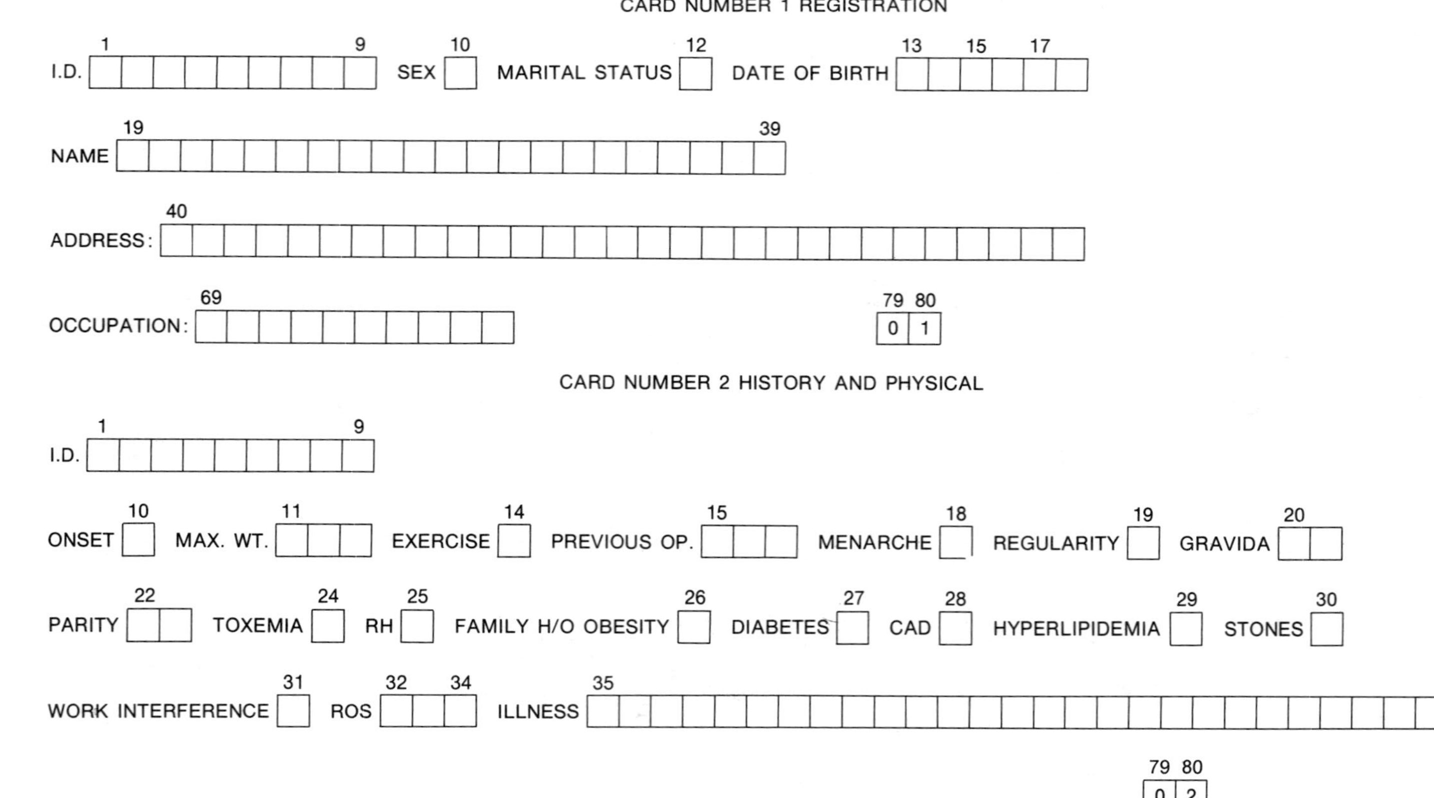

Figure 5.6 Data collection form for Project 5.2.

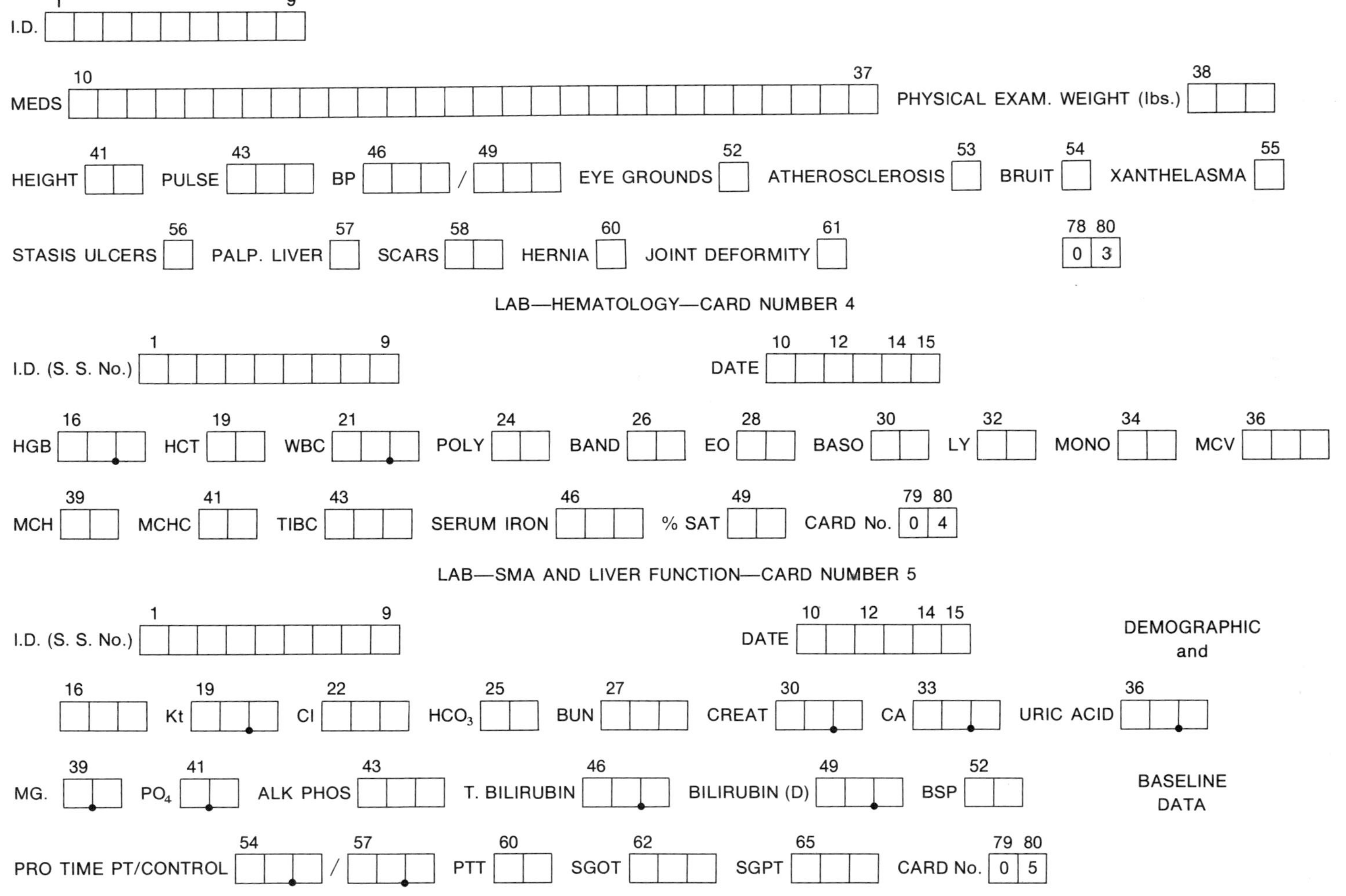

I.D. 1 … 9

MEDS 10 … 37 PHYSICAL EXAM. WEIGHT (lbs.) 38

HEIGHT 41 PULSE 43 BP 46 / 49 EYE GROUNDS 52 ATHEROSCLEROSIS 53 BRUIT 54 XANTHELASMA 55

STASIS ULCERS 56 PALP. LIVER 57 SCARS 58 HERNIA 60 JOINT DEFORMITY 61 78 80 [0 3]

LAB—HEMATOLOGY—CARD NUMBER 4

I.D. (S. S. No.) 1 … 9 DATE 10 12 14 15

HGB 16 HCT 19 WBC 21 POLY 24 BAND 26 EO 28 BASO 30 LY 32 MONO 34 MCV 36

MCH 39 MCHC 41 TIBC 43 SERUM IRON 46 % SAT 49 CARD No. 79 80 [0 4]

LAB—SMA AND LIVER FUNCTION—CARD NUMBER 5

I.D. (S. S. No.) 1 … 9 DATE 10 12 14 15

16 Kt 19 Cl 22 HCO_3 25 BUN 27 CREAT 30 CA 33 URIC ACID 36

MG. 39 PO_4 41 ALK PHOS 43 T. BILIRUBIN 46 BILIRUBIN (D) 49 BSP 52

PRO TIME PT/CONTROL 54 / 57 PTT 60 SGOT 62 SGPT 65 CARD No. 79 80 [0 5]

DEMOGRAPHIC and BASELINE DATA

Figure 5.6 (continued)

Table 5.1 Card 2 codes

Columns	*Measurement*
1–9	Social security number
10	History of onset of obesity first note at age of: 1. 0–5 yr 2. 5–10 yr 3. 10–15 yr 4. 15–25 yr 5. 25–40 yr 6. 40+ yr
11–13	Maximum weight, lb
14	Exercise tolerance: 1. tires rapidly on level ground 2. climb 1 flight of stairs 3. climb 2 flight of stairs 4. climb 3 flight of stairs
15–17	Previous operations: 1. small bowel bypass 2. take down of previous bypass 3. cholecystectomy 4. nephro- or ureterolithotomy 5. other
18	Onset of menarche: 1. 12–17 years of age 2. 18 or over years of age
19	Menstrual regularity: 1. premenarche 2. regular 3. hypo- or oligomenorrhoea 4. amenorrhoea 5. menopausal 6. postmenopausal
20–21	Gravida
22–23	Parity
24	History of Toxemia: 1. yes 2. no
25	History of Rh incompatibility 1. yes 2. no
26	Family history of obesity 1. yes 2. no

Table 5.1 (continued)

Columns	*Measurement*
27	Family history of diabetes mellitus 1. yes 2. no
28	Family history of coronary artery disease 1. yes 2. no
29	Family history of hyperlipidemia 1. yes 2. no
30	Family history of urinary stones 1. yes 2. no
31	Work interference 1. yes 2. no
32–34	Review of systems
35–63	Past history of illnesses 01. diabetes 02. hypertension 03. congestive heart failure 04. arteriosclerotic coronary artery disease 05. arteriosclerotic peripheral vascular disease 06. venous stasis ulcers 07. Pickwickian syndrome 08. cholecystitis 09. hepatitis 10. cirrhosis 11. transfusion reaction 12. adrenal disease 13. thyroid disease 14. nephro- or ureterolithiasis 15. gout 16. degenerative arthritis 17. hernia, ventral or inguinal 18. psychiatric disorder, depression 19. ulcer disease 20. other

Card 3 contains information about medications being taken and various physical conditions. The medication responses are reported in the same manner as were illnesses on the second card, in two column fields between columns 10 and 31. Columns 32 through 37 will be left blank. The codes for medications being taken and the remaining codes for the non-numerical responses are given in Table 5.2.

Cards 4 and 5 contain the results of various lab tests that are performed on each patient entering the study. Hemoglobin (HGB) is a number such as 14.3 or 12.9 for most people. Thus, three digits are required to code HGB properly, two whole digits and one digit after the decimal. Note that the decimal point is placed on the data collection form between the appropriate columns so that the person filling in the data will do so consistently for all people. *One key to the success of a data collection form is the consistency of the data coding.* The researcher also must be sure to provide enough columns to code the entire number adequately. For example, if it were possible for HGB to reach 100, the researcher could not code that high with the present format. When in doubt, you should always leave an extra column, because it is much better to have an unused column for insurance rather than not to have enough space. On cards 4 and 5, containing laboratory data, you can see clearly where columns were left to accommodate decimal points. These decimal points themselves are not actually keypunched, because the computer program written to manage the data can easily supply the decimal point. Also, if the HGB is 14, it should be coded as 14.0: that is, the decimal part of the number should be filled in with a zero. This procedure will minimize computer programming problems resulting from the fact that various programs would handle that blank column differently.

This complete form has three major components. The first component, of which part is presented here, represents presurgical baseline information. The second set contains data regarding the gastric partition surgery, and the third set contains postsurgery follow-up data. Some patients may have two sets of surgery data if a second surgery is performed, and all patients eventually have numerous sets of follow-up data collected after surgery.

This data collection form is long and complex, because measurements are collected over a period of time, and not all people have the same number of follow-up visits. However, this coding scheme is complete enough so that someone should be able to write a program that can read and collate this information as is necessary to carry out any statistical analyses. Note also that these forms were printed with the use of carbon triplicate. One form is included in the patient's medical record, one copy in files kept by the Department of Surgery, and the third copy is sent out for data processing. The additional printing cost for triplicate copies is a small price to pay for the insurance against loss of such a valuable data set.

Let us now look at another example to see a common type of problem that occurs often with data collection forms.

Table 5.2 Card 3 codes

Columns	*Measurement*
10–37	Present medicines: 01. insulin 02. oral hypoglycemics 03. atromid-S 04. other hypolipemics 05. digoxin 06. aldomet 07. hydrochlorthiagide 08. hydralogine 09. reserpine 10. guanethidine 11. others
52	Diabetic eye grounds 1. yes 2. no
54	Bruits: 1. yes 2. no
55	Xauthalasma: 1. yes 2. no
56	Stasis ulcers: 1. yes 2. no
57	Palp lines: 1. yes 2. no
58–59	Scars: 1. upper midline 2. paramedian 3. transverse 4. right subcostal 5. other
60	Hernia: 1. ventral 2. inguinal
61	Joint deformity: 1. yes 2. no

5.5 COMMON PROBLEMS WITH CODING SCHEMES

Refer to Project 5.1, where a data collection form was designed to collect information about the drug usage of mentally retarded people at a government center. The researcher has been collecting data now for some time, and a few problems have arisen. One problem is in the dosing interval (DI) code. A single column was allocated to this response, and nine possible outcomes were coded. During data collection, it has become obvious that the defined categories are not satisfactory to describe adequately all possible dosing intervals. The same problem has occurred with the codes for route of administration. Also, because this project is being carried out over a long period of time and there is a large turnover in the doctors serving this center, the two-digit code for the doctor prescribing each drug is inadequate.

How can these problems be resolved at this point in the research project? The form cannot be changed now unless the researcher wishes to redesign it completely and treat the total collection of data as two separate data sets. Of course, computer programs could be written to combine the data sets and answer the appropriate questions that will be raised. However, this approach would require much more work in the data management part of the project, and there may be a simpler means of resolving the problem.

Consider using the same codes as already defined for DI, but adding to them the following codes.

Further drug codes

Code	*Unit Doses*	*Administered*
A	3	Once daily
B	4	Once daily
C	2	Every 4 hr
D	1	once weekly
E	1	twice weekly
F	1	3 times weekly
G	2	once weekly
H	2	twice weekly
I	2	3 times weekly
J	3	twice daily
K	3	twice weekly
L	4	3 times weekly
M	$\frac{1}{2}$	twice daily
N	4	twice weekly
O	1	every 4 hr
P	$\frac{1}{2}$	daily
Q	4	twice daily
R	$\frac{1}{2}$	twice daily

The following codes could be added to the route response:

A	vaginal
B	buccal
C	sublingual
D	intra-articular
E	intradermal
F	introperitoneal

Doctors entering the study after 99 have been coded could be identified as A, B, C, . . . , Z, then AA, AB, AC, . . . , AZ, and so on.

In each of these situations, we have stayed within the allowable columns by using letters of the alphabet as codes. This approach is perfectly appropriate as long as the computer program written to manage the data can be changed. This change is simple in some computer systems and difficult in others. Although in this project we were able to resolve the problem fairly easily, *you should adequately code all the responses before data collection begins*.

Note that the number zero has not been used as a code for a qualitative response in any of our examples. The reason is that various computer program packages have different ways of handling blank values. Some packages do not distinguish between a blank column and a code of zero unless certain statements are included to prevent this ambiguity. Thus, if you do not know how the chosen computer program handles this situation, erroneous results can occur. It is best to avoid using zero as a code. If the computer package distinguishes between blanks and zeroes or if the person responsible for the data management knows how to use the available program to get around this situation, there should be no problem. You should *not* decide to use zero as a code because you do not expect any missing data. Problems often arise that lead to missing data. Even the most optimistic researcher should be wary of missing data and, hence, of using zero as a code.

In Chapter 6 we shall look at another type of data collection form, a questionnaire type that is filled out by many individuals. This data collection form also should be designed in such a way as to minimize the time and errors in data processing.

5.6 KEY POINTS

Many benefits are derived from designing a data collection form before beginning the collection of your research data. If you are submitting a grant proposal, it will show the granting agency that you have carefully considered the data to collect and a form for accurately reporting it. A proper data collection form ensures that your data will not have to be transcribed; hence, transcription errors will be avoided. Finally, a well-designed data collection form simplifies data processing. The result is faster processing with fewer errors, which means lower processing cost.

The categories of data to be processed are demographic information, extraneous factor levels, factor levels, and response variable measurements. In each category, each recorded response is either categorical or numerical. For each numerical measurement, the appropriate number of spaces must be allocated to fill in the number. The decimal point, if needed, should be included between the appropriate spaces. Categorical measurements can be coded as either numerical or alphamerical depending on your preference and available statistical software.

A particular type of data collection form is a questionnaire to have people fill out. Because many people will be completing these forms, you must be certain that questions are clearly stated, possible responses are comprehensive, and responses are coded so that the completed forms can be processed. Chapter 6 presents rules for questionnaire design.

CHAPTER 6

Designing a Questionnaire

6.1 INTRODUCTION

Questionnaire data are different from those we have seen. The data forms are filled out by the people participating in the study rather than by researchers. Thus, if you hope to have this form keypunched directly, the questionnaire (and data collection form) must be laid out in such a way that 1) the respondent can clearly mark all appropriate answers and 2) the keypunchers can easily follow the flow of the form and know which responses are coded in which columns.

6.2 THE IDEAL QUESTIONNAIRE

Let us look at an example of a well-designed questionnaire.

Project 6.1 Toothpaste comparison study

Refer to Project 3.4, whose objective was **to compare a new toothpaste (Brand A) to three other commercial brands of toothpaste (Brand B, Brand C, and Brand D) for flavor acceptance and gingivitis control.**

Before entering this study, each participant is asked to fill out a dental health and background questionnaire. A copy of that form is shown in Figure 6.1. Note that the questions are spaced far enough apart so that the respondent has enough room to mark the answer clearly and the keypuncher

Name ______________

Subject Identification ____
(1–4)

Product Code ____
(6)

Site ____
(8–9)

DENTAL HEALTH AND BACKGROUND QUESTIONNAIRE

1. Your age at last birthday ______________ 11–1
2. Please indicate sex (circle one) M F 13
3. Please rate your general physical health as 14
   1. Excellent 2. Good 3. Fair 4. Poor
4. Have you had any serious illness during the past year? 15
   1. Yes 2. No
5. If yes, did you lose considerable time (10 days or more) from school or work? 16
   1. Yes 2. No
6. I would rate my *oral* health as 17
   1. Excellent 2. Good
7. Are any of your teeth capped or crowned? 18
   1. Yes 2. No
8. If yes, how many are capped or crowned? ______________ 19–20
9. Do you visit your dentist regularly (at least every 6 months)? 21
   1. Yes 2. No
10. I have had one of the following: cold sores, blisters, canker sores or ulcers in my mouth or on my lips. 22
    1. Once every two months 2. Once or twice a year 3. Never
11. I have experienced cracking at the corners of the mouth and at the edge of my lips. 23
    1. Once every two months 2. Once or twice a year 3. Never
12. Do you have the habit of biting your cheek, lips or tongue? 25
    1. Yes 2. No
13. I have had the following dental conditions over the past year.

	Frequently 1	Occasionally 2	Never 3	
a. Cavities	____	____	____	26
b. Gums bleed easily	____	____	____	27
c. Gums feel sore	____	____	____	28
d. It hurts to chew	____	____	____	29
e. Cold food/drinks bother my teeth	____	____	____	30
f. Hot foods/drinks bother my teeth	____	____	____	31
g. Sweet foods/drinks bother my teeth	____	____	____	32
h. Tartar builds up on my teeth	____	____	____	33

14. Do you use a mouthwash? 34
    1. Frequently 2. Occasionally 3. Never
15. Which mouthwash do you use? 35
    1. Listerine 3. Lavoris
    2. Scope 4. Other. Name brand ______________
16. Do you brush your teeth? 36
    1. Less than once per day 4. Three times a day
    2. Once a day 5. Four times a day
    3. Twice a day 6. More than four times a day

Figure 6.1 Demographic and dental health information.

17. I brush my teeth with my — 37
    1. Right Hand 2. Left Hand
18. What toothpaste do you usually use? (circle one) — 38
    1. Crest (either flavor) 6. Aim
    2. Colgate MFP 7. Pepsodent
    3. Gleem II 8. Red Close-Up
    4. Ultra brite 9. Green Close-Up
    5. Macleans (either flavor) 10. Other. Name brand ______________
19. Do you use breath fresheners? — 40
    1. No 2. Yes
20. Which brand do you usually use? Circle one: — 41
    1. Certs 3. Other. Name brand ______________
    2. Clorets
21. Do you chew gum? If so, circle flavor. — 42
    1. Peppermint 4. Fruit
    2. Spearmint 5. Other (name flavor) ______________
    3. Cinnamon 6. Never chew gum
22. What primary reason influences your choice of toothpaste? (circle one) — 43
    1. Decay fighting 5. Parents make choice
    2. Whitening 6. Flavor
    3. Cleaning 7. Other
    4. Breath freshening
23. Do you have any allergies? — 44
    1. Yes 2. No
24. If yes, please indicate below
    1. Dust — 45
    2. Animal hair — 46
    3. Rose fever — 47
    4. Certain foods or beverages Name item ______________ — 48
    5. Certain candies or gum Name item ______________ — 49
    6. Certain toothpastes or mouthwashes Name item ______________ — 50
    7. After-shaves or perfumes Name item ______________ — 51
    8. Certain drugs or medicines Name item ______________ — 52
    9. Cosmetics Name item ______________ — 53
    10. Other Name item ______________ — 54

Figure 6.1 (Continued)

can follow this questionnaire easily. Also, for the keypuncher's benefit, the columns have been coded on the right edge of the form. This form is laid out in such a straightforward manner that it needs virtually no added description. Only question 18 needs an explanation of its code. A single column has been allocated for the type of toothpaste used, but *other* is coded as 10. For keypunching, it would be coded as a zero. Otherwise, it should be left blank. This data collection form is ideal for both the respondent and the keypuncher.

6.3 PROBLEMS IN DESIGNING QUESTIONNAIRES

A much less than ideal form for a questionnaire is provided in Figure 6.2. This questionnaire poses so many problems for both the respondent and the

Name: Date of birth: Age:
Address: Phone number:
Name of close friend who lives locally:
Address of above:
Name of closest living relative:
Address of above:
How long have you been a resident of Florida?
Where did you reside the major portion of your life?

Family history:

A

Father:
If deceased, age at time of death? . . . . ______
Cause of death, if definitely known. If unknown, please state so ______

______

Did he have high blood pressure?	Yes	No	Unknown
Did he have heart trouble?	Yes	No	Unknown
Did he have rheumatic heart trouble?	Yes	No	Unknown
Did he have hardening of the arteries to the brain?	Yes	No	Unknown
Did he have poor circulation to the lower limbs?	Yes	No	Unknown
Did he have definitely known diabetes mellitus?	Yes	No	Unknown
Did he smoke cigarettes?	Yes	No	Unknown

If the answer to the last question was yes, about how many a day? ______
Again, if the answer to the previous question was yes, how many years did he smoke? . . . . ______

Did he take medication for any of the above? Yes No Unknown
If the answer is yes, then for which one of the conditions? ______
Do you know the name of the medication? If so please give the name, if not please state "unknown" ______
Was, or is, your father overweight? Yes No Unknown
If yes, would you say slight, moderate or severe? ______

Mother:
If deceased, age at time of death? . . . . ______
Cause of death, if definitely known. If unknown, please state so ______

______

Did she have high blood pressure?	Yes	No	Unknown
Did she have heart trouble?	Yes	No	Unknown
Did she have rheumatic heart trouble?	Yes	No	Unknown
Did she have hardening of the arteries to the brain?	Yes	No	Unknown
Did she have poor circulation to the lower limbs?	Yes	No	Unknown
Did she have definitely known diabetes mellitus?	Yes	No	Unknown
Did she smoke cigarettes?	Yes	No	Unknown

If the answer to the last question was yes, about how many a day? ______
Again, if the answer to the last question was yes, how many years did she smoke? . . . . ______

Did she take medication for any of the above? Yes No Unknown
If the answer is yes, then for which of the conditions? ______
Do you know the name of the medication? If so please give the name, if not please state "unknown" ______
Was, or is, your mother overweight? Yes No Unknown
If yes, would you state slight, moderate or severe? ______

Figure 6.2 Poorly designed questionnaire.

Other family:
Do you have any living brothers? Yes No
If the answer is yes, how many? . . . . ________
Do any of them have high blood pressure? Yes No Unknown
If the answer is definitely yes, how many? ________

B {
Do they, or does he, take medication for the same? Yes No Unknown
If they do take medication, do you know the name of this? ________
How long have they been taking it? . . . . ________
What is the name of the medication, if known? ________
}

Did he or they have heart trouble? Yes No Unknown
Did he or they have hardening of the arteries to the brain? Yes No Unknown
Did he or they have poor circulation to the lower limbs? Yes No Unknown
Did he or they have diabetes mellitus? Yes No Unknown
Did he or they have high cholesterol? Yes No Unknown
Did he or they smoke cigarettes? Yes No Unknown
If yes, for approximately how many years did he smoke and how many did he smoke a day?
____
Was he, or were they, overweight? Yes No Unknown
Do you have any living sisters? Yes No
If the answer is yes, how many? . . . . ________
Do any of them have high blood pressure? Yes No Unknown
If the answer is definitely yes, how many? ________
Do they, or does she, take medication for the same? Yes No Unknown
If they do take medication, do you know the name of this? Yes No
How long have they been taking it? . . . . ________
What is the name of the medication, if known? ________
Did she or they have heart trouble? Yes No Unknown
Did she or they ever have hardening of the arteries to the brain? Yes No Unknown
Did she or they have poor circulation to the lower limbs? Yes No Unknown
Did she or they have diabetes mellitus? Yes No Unknown
Did she or they have high cholesterol? Yes No Unknown
Did she or they smoke cigarettes? Yes No Unknown
If yes, for approximately how many years did she smoke and how many did she smoke a day?
____
Was she, or were they, overweight? Yes No Unknown

C {
Have any brothers expired? Yes No If expired, age at death? ________
Have any sisters expired? Yes No If expired, age at death? ________
}

Do you have frequent headaches? Yes No
If yes, are they located in the front, back, sides, right, left, both? (Please circle appropriate answer.)
Do they usually occur at a particular time of the day? Yes No
If the answer is yes, then approximately what time; that is, in the morning, mid-day, afternoon, or night?
Do you have frequent episodes of lightheadedness, with lightheadedness being defined as a feeling of near-fainting or "floating"? Yes No
Do you have episodes of dizziness, with dizziness being defined as episodes where either you or your surroundings spin around? Yes No
Do you have ringing in your ears? Yes No
If the answer to the ringing in the ears is yes, is this constant or infrequent? Yes No
One ear or both ears? (Please circle appropriate answer) Yes No
Do you have transient episodes of loss of vision, in either one or both eyes? Yes No

Figure 6.2 (Continued)

Have you ever had any problem relative to your eyes, that you have been told by your ophthalmologist (eye doctor) is attributable to some systemic disease? Yes No

If the answer is yes, then what disease? ______

Have you ever been told by your eye doctor that you have changes in your eyes that reflect high blood pressure? Yes No

Have you ever been told by your eye doctor that you have changes in your eyes that reflect hardening of the arteries? Yes No

When did you have your last eye examination by an ophthalmologist, that is, an eye doctor?

______

Do you have definitely known heart trouble? Yes No

If the answer is yes, please circle the appropriate description that follows.

Have had definite coronary thrombosis, myocardial infarction, or an attack or damage to my heart.

Have had enlarged heart.

Have had heart irregularity.

Have had rheumatic heart disease.

Have had leaky valve, injured valve or scarred valve.

Have had heart failure, lungs filling with fluid, or liver enlargement because my heart was not working as it should.

Have you ever been told of poor circulation to your legs or feet? Yes No

If yes, how has this manifested itself? Please circle the appropriate answer below:

Feet cold.

Pain in calves of legs with walking that goes away when I stop and rest, but returns when I resume walking.

Discomfort with exposure to cold.

Discoloration with exposure to cold.

Figure 6.2 (Continued)

keypuncher that it is difficult even to know where to begin pointing them out. It would be virtually impossible to keypunch this form as it currently stands. The questions are bunched so closely together that a keypuncher could not possibly follow it without missing some answers, especially if the respondent left any answers blank. Also, the keypuncher has no idea which responses are to go in which columns.

Let us point out a few of the problems with this questionnaire. They are not the only ones, but they indicate the poor quality of the entire questionnaire. Since the questions are not even numbered, we shall mark each question to be discussed.

Let us begin with family history responses (A). A line is left for the age at which the father died. However, it is not marked as to what columns age goes into or how many columns are allocated. Three columns should be left for age, because it is conceivable that the age of death is over 100. The next question asks the respondent to list the cause of death. The question, as stated, is open ended, requiring the respondent to write in the cause of death. An open-ended question like this cannot be computerized directly but would require the researcher to code the cause of death into categories. To save this work, the categories of interest should be given on the questionnaire. The respondent then can choose the most appropriate category. Here is one possible set of codes for this question:

1. Liver disease
2. Heart disease
3. Cancer
4. Pneumonia, meningitis, or other infectious disease
5. Diabetes or other endocrine disease
6. Accident or injury
7. Suicide
8. Other
9. Unknown

This format would make the question closed ended and provide more useful information if the researcher can identify all appropriate categories.

Each of the next few questions has a categorical response. The code that will be used for each response also should be printed to assist the keypuncher. For example, the format

1. Yes 2. No 3. Unknown

would provide the code and reduce the number of errors made by the keypunchers.

One question asks how many cigarettes the father smoked per day. If the number 2 appeared as the answer, it would not be clear whether that 2 referred to two cigarettes or to two packs of cigarettes. The answer should be listed as

__ cigarettes per day.

This format would make it clear to the respondent exactly how the question should be answered.

The next set of questions, concerning medications for the above mentioned illnesses, cannot be adequately answered by the respondent as they are stated and, hence will provide no relevant information to the researcher. The questions should be either removed from the questionnaire or rewritten to produce the desired responses. The major problem with these questions is that only one medication can be listed for one of the listed illnesses. To get the desired information, the researcher should have stated the questions as follows:

1. Did he have high blood pressure? 1. Yes 2. No 3. Unknown

2. If yes, did he take medication for this?	1. Yes	2. No	3. Unknown
3. If yes, do you know the name of the medication? If not, please state unknown.	1. Yes	2. No	3. Unknown

This series of questions should be repeated for each of the remaining five illnesses listed.

The last question concerning father's medical history should be stated as follows:

If yes, was overweight condition
1. slight
2. moderate
3. severe

As the question is stated currently, the keypuncher would not be able to code the answer.

In section B of the questionnaire, the questions provide no useful information to the researcher. If more than one brother has high blood pressure, these questions can provide the information for only one brother. Likewise, for section C, space is provided to list only one age of death, yet more than one sibling may have died.

The questions and answers on the questionnaire are bunched so closely that both the respondent and the keypuncher would have a hard time reading them. The questions should be spaced farther apart, with the possible responses coded and listed either below or to the right of the questions. A clearer statement of these questions is shown in Figure 6.3.

6.4 MORE DESIGN CONSIDERATIONS

If you want most respondents to cooperate in answering a questionnaire, it must look appealing to them. First, print on both sides of a sheet of paper. In this way a four-page questionnaire is contained on two sheets of paper. People are discouraged by a lot of paper, so keep the number of sheets to a minimum.

Avoid asking irrelevant or repetitious questions. Readers become disinterested if they feel that questions are wasting their time. As a result, the questionnaire is not completed or returned.

Sometimes it is advised that certain questions be restated in a different form and included a second time in the questionnaire. The main reason is to

PERSONAL HISTORY

59. Do you have frequent headaches? 1. Yes 2. No 3. Unknown

---

60. If yes, are they located in the
    1. Front
    2. Back
    3. Right
    4. Left
    5. All over
    6. None of above

---

61. Do they usually occur at a particular time of the day? 1. Yes 2. No 3. Unknown

---

62. If yes, are they usually in the
    1. Morning
    2. Afternoon
    3. Night
    4. No particular time

---

63. Do you have frequent episodes of light-headedness, with this being defined as a feeling of near fainting or floating? 1. Yes 2. No 3. Unknown
64. Do you have episodes of dizziness, with dizziness being defined as episodes where either you or your surroundings are spinning around? 1. Yes 2. No 3. Unknown
65. Are either of the above brought on by changing your position? 1. Yes 2. No 3. Unknown
66. Do you have ringing or buzzing in your ears? 1. Yes 2. No 3. Unknown
67. If the answer to the latter is yes, is this constant? 1. Yes 2. No 3. Unknown
68. Do you have episodes of "blacking out" (i.e., loss of consciousness and falling to the floor)? 1. Yes 2. No 3. Unknown
69. Have you had any episodes of brief loss of speech? 1. Yes 2. No 3. Unknown
70. Have you had a period of brief loss of use of your arm or leg or both? 1. Yes 2. No 3. Unknown
71. Have you had episodes of numbness involving one arm or one leg or both one arm and one leg? 1. Yes 2. No 3. Unknown
72. Have you ever had a stroke? 1. Yes 2. No 3. Unknown
73. Have you had more than one stroke? 1. Yes 2. No 3. Unknown
74. Do you have episodes of transient loss of vision in either one or both eyes? 1. Yes 2. No 3. Unknown
75. Have you had any problem with your eyes that a doctor has said might be caused by a general health problem? 1. Yes 2. No 3. Unknown
76. Have you ever been told by a doctor that you have changes in your eyes caused by high blood pressure? 1. Yes 2. No 3. Unknown
77. Have you ever been told by a doctor that you have changes in your eyes caused by hardening of the arteries? 1. Yes 2. No 3. Unknown

---

78. When did you have your last eye examination by an ophthalmologist?
    1. Within last year
    2. 1–2 years
    3. More than 2 years

---

79. Do you have any chest discomfort with exercise or physical effort? 1. Yes 2. No 3. Unknown
80. Do you have any chest discomfort with tension or anxiety? 1. Yes 2. No 3. Unknown

Figure 6.3 A better format for the questionnaire in Figure 6.2.

determine the consistency of the respondent by comparing his or her responses to the same question. If the same person's answers differ to a question asked two times, you may not place much confidence in any of his or her answers.

However, if you decide to repeat questions, be extremely careful to do it so that the respondent does not perceive it. If respondents notice that questions are repeated, they will feel either that you are trying to trick them or that you are wasting their time. In either case, your questionnaire probably will not be returned. To maximize the response rate, you must eliminate as many reasons as possible why people will not respond.

Have your peers review your questionnaire before you use it for questions that may be irrelevant or unclear. Also, a small pilot study of respondents can provide a great deal of information as to whether there are unforeseen problems with your questionnaire.

Use closed-ended questions rather than open-ended questions. An example of such a question stated both ways is given below.

What is your attitude toward abortion?

____

____

____

____

____

or

What is your attitude toward abortion?

____ 1. I believe in abortion for any woman who wants it.
____ 2. I believe abortion should be allowed in certain instances.
____ 3. I am undecided concerning my attitude toward abortion.
____ 4. I am totally opposed to abortion.

The first example is an open-ended statement: the respondent has the freedom to answer the question in as much detail as he or she desires. In the second example, the closed-ended statement simply allows the respondent to check the category that most closely reflects his or her feelings.

The open-ended question has two shortcomings. First, if a potential respondent scans the questionnaire and sees many open-ended questions, he or she may decide that too much is being asked or that the questionnaire will take too much time to complete. The result will be no response from that person. A second shortcoming is that an open-ended response will have to be categorized or quantified by the researcher in the data analysis. The researcher would have to feel confident that the respondent's answer is interpreted correctly. One possible solution to this problem is the closed-ended question. It has the disadvantage that it may stifle the respondent, but if carefully thought out, it should cover all possible responses adequately. If you are afraid of omitting a possible response, the catch-all category of *Other*, followed by room to elaborate, can be added to the list of responses to each question.

References 1 and 2 provide excellent discussions on questionnaire design.

6.5 A MAIL-OUT QUESTIONNAIRE

Let us look at a good example of a mail-out questionnaire. (This project is presented by permission of Paul L. Doerring, Associate Professor; Dr. William C. McCormick, Associate Professor; Deborah L. Klapp, Adjunct Clinical Instructor; and Dr. Wayne L. Russell, Clinical Practitioner, all of the College of Pharmacy, University of Florida.)

Project 6.2 Example of a mail-out questionnaire

This study was a national survey of hospital pharmacists concerning non-chemically equivalent drug product substitution. The four-page questionnaire of 34 questions, shown in Figure 6.4, was printed on a single 11 by 17 in. sheet and folded. A light brown paper was chosen along with dark brown ink to give the questionnaire a more pleasing and professional look. Note that questions requiring numerical responses, such as questions 4 and 8, provide the appropriate number of spaces and an example showing the respondent how to fill in the spaces. Where questions allow multiple responses, such as in question 11, an asterisk (*) appears in front of the question. This notation serves a dual purpose, reminding the respondent that multiple responses are allowed and alerting the data processors that more than one response may be given. For question 10, where only one response is allowed, the data processor would place a 1 or 2 in the column assigned to that question. For question 11, four columns are designated, and a 1 is placed in the column for each of the responses checked. The remaining columns in the set of four are left blank. Thus, if a participant checked both 1 and 2 for question 11, the keypuncher would punch 1 1 B B (where B denotes the column left blank) in the four columns used for question 11. Some researchers may decide not to leave any columns blank, instead coding zero if the response was not checked.

Finally, note that all questions that have many categories to choose from also include a category *other,* along with space to elaborate. This choice is provided in case there is an important category that the researchers overlooked in designing the questionnaire.

SURVEY OF NON-CHEMICALLY EQUIVALENT DRUG PRODUCT SUBSTITUTION IN HOSPITALS

This survey has been sent to all short-term hospitals in the United States. Responses will be strictly anonymous. Please take approximately 15 minutes to answer the following questions. Definitions are included to make clear our meaning. Certain questions may have more than one answer and are indicated by an asterisk and the words **"Check all that apply."** Otherwise, please check only one answer.

1. What best describes the ownership of your institution?

☐ 1. Government, Non federal, City
☐ 2. Government, Non federal, County
☐ 3. Government, Nonfederal, State
☐ 4. Government, Federal
☐ 5. Nongovernment, nonprofit, church-operated
☐ 6. Nongovernment, nonprofit, and not church-operated.
☐ 7. Investor-owned (Private, for-profit)

2. Is your institution a teaching hospital affiliated with a medical school?

☐ 1. Yes
☐ 2. No

3. In what state is your hospital located? ______________________________

____ ____

4. What is the number of beds? (**Example:** 0 3 4 0 for 340 beds)

____ ____ ____ ____

5. How many advanced degree (Pharm.D., M.S., or Ph.D.) pharmacists does your hospital pharmacy employ?

____ ____

6. Is your hospital an accredited ASHP residency site?

☐ 1. Yes
☐ 2. No

7. Do you have a unit dose system of drug distribution? **Definition:** *Unit dose distribution = almost all drugs dispensed in a single dose unit package in an amount not exceeding a 24 hour supply.*

☐ 1. Yes
☐ 2. No

8. What percent of your hospital beds are served in this way? (**Example:** 0 8 5 % for 85 percent)

____ ____ ____%

9. Do pharmacy personnel participate in development of criteria for patient care audits or collect and analyze drug use data for presentation to physicians?

☐ 1. Yes
☐ 2. No

10. Is a formulary system in operation in your hospital?

☐ 1. Yes
☐ 2. No

If no, go to question 13.

*11. Does each physician give **prior** general consent to operation of the formulary system by: (**check all that apply**) **Definition:** *Prior Consent = authorization prior to the writing of the order.*

☐ 1. Signing a statement to abide by the hospital bylaws upon admission to the medical staff.
☐ 2. Giving prior consent expressed in a separate document describing the formulary system.
☐ 3. Prior consent not obtained.
☐ 4. Other ______________________________

* More than one response can be given.

12. Does each physician give **current** consent by the use of a suitably worded imprint on medication order forms? **Example:** *Some form of the statement "Formulary equivalent will be dispensed unless otherwise indicated."*

☐ 1. Yes
☐ 2. No

Figure 6.4 Questionnaire for a national survey.

13. Does your formulary system and/or drug distribution system allow selection and automatic dispensing of a single drug product in the case of multiple-source, **chemical equivalents**? **Example:** *Only one brand of Ampicillin is stocked and dispensed regardless of the trade name ordered.*

☐ 1. Yes
☐ 2. No

14. Does your formulary system and/or drug distribution system allow **stocking** of a single, therapeutic equivalent drug product in a class? **Definition:** *Therapeutic equivalent is a product chosen to represent a class and is therapeutically but not chemically equivalent to other drugs in the class.* **Example:** *Stocking cephradine as the only oral cephalosporin on the formulary.*

☐ 1. Yes
☐ 2. No

If answer is no, skip to question 17.

*15. How are physicians informed when the Pharmacy and Therapeutics Committee has first selected a single, therapeutically but not chemically equivalent drug product to represent a class? (**Check all that apply**).

☐ 1. One time notification via letter, memorandum, or newsletter, etc. circulated to medical staff.
☐ 2. Periodic notification (more than once) via letter, memorandum, or newsletter, etc. circulated to medical staff.
☐ 3. Printed in formulary or medical staff manual.
☐ 4. No notification of this decision.
☐ 5. Other ______________________

16. Does the operation of your formulary system allow **automatic** dispensing of the therapeutically equivalent drug product without contacting the prescribing physician for his permission? **Example:** *When an order for cephalexin is received, cephradine is dispensed since cephradine has been chosen as the only oral cephalosporin on the formulary.*

☐ 1. Yes
☐ 2. No

If yes, skip to question 18.

*17. Since your formulary system and/or drug distribution system does **not** allow automatic dispensing of a therapeutic equivalent, which of the following describe the reason(s) for not allowing this? (**Check all that apply**)

☐ 1. It violates state and/or federal laws.
☐ 2. It would not be accepted by the physicians practicing in our hospital.
☐ 3. Unnecessary risk of civil liability (risk of law suit) is assumed by those determining therapeutic equivalency.
☐ 4. It interferes with the physician's right to select the drug which is, in his opinion, best suited for the patient.
☐ 5. The expected benefits do not justify the costs involved in setting up and maintaining such a system.
☐ 6. We have not thought about this type of exchange.
☐ 7. Other ______________________

Skip to question 30

*18. How are physicians informed of the interchange of the **therapeutic equivalent** after they have written the order? (**Check all that apply**)

☐ 1. Written notification from pharmacy which becomes a permanent part of the patient's medical record.
☐ 2. Written notification from pharmacy which is not a permanent part of the medical record (i.e., attached to the outside of the chart, nurses' kardex, etc.)
☐ 3. Verbal notification.
☐ 4. None of the above.
☐ 5. Other ______________________

* More than one response can be given.

19. Is this notification of interchange provided:

☐ 1. Before the therapeutic equivalent is dispensed but after the order is written?
☐ 2. Within 24 hours of the first dose of the therapeutic equivalent dispensed?
☐ 3. After 24 hours but during the course of therapy?
☐ 4. Not notified during course of therapy?

20. Was consideration of the potential for legal challenge an important factor in developing the notification procedures indicated in questions #18 and #19.

☐ 1. Yes
☐ 2. No

Figure 6.4 (Continued)

21. How aware do you feel the physician is that an interchange of **therapeutic equivalents** has taken place?

☐ 1. Aware all of the time.
☐ 2. Aware most of the time.
☐ 3. Aware less than half of the time.
☐ 4. Rarely aware.
☐ 5. Not able to estimate.

22. How often does the Medication Administration Record accurately reflect the actual brand or generic name administered after an interchange of **therapeutic equivalents** has taken place?

☐ 1. All of the time.
☐ 2. Most of the time.
☐ 3. Less than half of the time.
☐ 4. Rarely.
☐ 5. Not able to estimate.

23. How often does the pharmacy profile card accurately reflect the actual brand or generic name after an interchange of **therapeutic equivalents** has occurred?

☐ 1. All of the time.
☐ 2. Most of the time.
☐ 3. Less than half of the time.
☐ 4. Rarely.
☐ 5. Not able to estimate.

*24. Which of the following persons play(s) a **significant** role(s) in deciding which product is therapeutically but not chemically equivalent to other drug products in a class? (see question #14 for an example.) (**Check all that apply.**)

☐ 1. Physicians serving on pharmacy and therapeutics committee.
☐ 2. Pharmacists serving on pharmacy and therapeutics committee.
☐ 3. Nurses serving on pharmacy and therapeutics committee.
☐ 4. Other physicians.
☐ 5. Other pharmacists.
☐ 6. Other nurses.
☐ 7. Other personnel, please specify ______________________

25. The person(s) **most** likely to be held primarily responsible in a civil action for interchange of a therapeutic equivalent is/are: (**Check only one**)

☐ 1. Executive committee of medical staff.
☐ 2. Director of Pharmacy.
☐ 3. Chief of the medical staff.
☐ 4. Hospital administrator.
☐ 5. Board of Trustees of the hospital.
☐ 6. Prescribing physician.
☐ 7. Dispensing pharmacist.
☐ 8. P&T Committee members.
☐ 9. Other ______________________

*26. The classes of drugs, for which a single **therapeutically equivalent** drug product **has** been selected is/are: (**Check all that apply**)

☐ A. Oral vitamins
☐ B. Oral antacids
☐ C. Antihistamines
☐ D. Benzodiazepines
☐ E. Cephalosporins, injectable
☐ F. Cephalosporins, oral
☐ G. Aminoglycosides
☐ H. Laxatives
☐ I. Barbiturates
☐ J. Other ______________________
____

*27. The following were important considerations in selecting the classes you indicated in question #26. Indicate the classes to which the consideration applied by placing the corresponding letter from #26 in the spaces to the right. **Example:** *If oral antacids were selected because of heavy use, put a "B" in one of the spaces for statement #1 below.*

1. Heavy use and high expenditures for drugs within the class. ___ ___ ___ ___ ___ ___
2. Great number of different chemical entities within the class. ___ ___ ___ ___ ___ ___
3. Physician interest in promoting rational therapy (i.e., willingness to analyze class category). ___ ___ ___ ___ ___ ___
4. Other ______________________ ___ ___ ___ ___ ___ ___

*28. The following were considerations in selecting which **drug product** represents the classes you indicated in question #26. Indicate the classes to which the considerations applied by placing the letter from #26 in the spaces to the right. **Example:** *If Maalox was selected as the oral antacid product because of its price, put a "B" in one of the spaces for statement #5 below.*

1. Promotional activity by manufacturer's representatives. ___ ___ ___ ___ ___ ___
2. Pharmacokinetic equivalency data (bioavailability, half-life, tissue levels, etc.). ___ ___ ___ ___ ___ ___
3. Clinical effectiveness equivalency data. ___ ___ ___ ___ ___ ___
4. Package insert indication equivalency. ___ ___ ___ ___ ___ ___
5. Price of the product. ___ ___ ___ ___ ___ ___
6. Services provided by the company (education, handling of back-orders, funding of studies, etc.).

Figure 6.4 (Continued)

7. Experience with availability of drugs from the company. ___ ___ ___ ___ ___ ___
8. Returned goods policy of the company. ___ ___ ___ ___ ___ ___
9. Experience with the quality of drugs from the company. ___ ___ ___ ___ ___ ___

29. What would you estimate the dollar value of yearly cost savings resulting from selection of therapeutically equivalent products to be?

☐ 1. $______________.
☐ 2. Cannot estimate but thought to be significant.
☐ 3. Cannot estimate but thought to be insignificant.

30. A bid system of purchasing is applied to what percent of your high use drugs? **Example:** 0 5 0 % *for 50 percent.*

___ ___ ___%

31. What would you estimate the dollar value of yearly cost savings resulting from bid purchasing of multisource **generic** equivalents (**chemical equivalents**) to be?

☐ 1. $______________.
☐ 2. Cannot estimate but thought to be significant.
☐ 3. Cannot estimate but thought to be insignificant.

*32. What **classes** of drugs are likely to be considered but are **not presently** represented by a single therapeutic equivalent? (**Check all that apply**).

☐ 1. Oral vitamins
☐ 2. Oral antacids
☐ 3. Antihistamines
☐ 4. Benzodiazepines
☐ 5. Cephalosporins, injectable
☐ 6. Cephalosporins, oral
☐ 7. Aminoglycosides
☐ 8. Laxatives
☐ 9. Barbiturates
☐ 10. Other ______________
☐ 11. No such action is likely.

33. How do you feel the Board of Pharmacy in your state would view the interchange of **non-chemically** but therapeutically equivalent drug products through the operation of a hospital formulary system?

☐ 1. Completely within state and/or federal law.
☐ 2. In accordance with policies and procedures established by the pharmacy and therapeutics committee and hence not subject to state or federal regulations.
☐ 3. In violation of state and/or federal laws.

*34. In terms of civil liability (risk of law suits) arising as a result of the interchange of **non-chemically** but therapeutically equivalent drug products, do you feel that such interchanges would: (**Check all that apply**).

☐ 1. Increase the liability of the prescribing physician.
☐ 2. Increase the liability of the person or persons determining therapeutic equivalency.
☐ 3. Increase the liability of the person or persons dispensing the product.
☐ 4. Increase the liability of the person administering the medication.
☐ 5. Increase the liability of the hospital.
☐ 6. Not likely to increase the risk of civil liability at all.
☐ 7. Have not thought about it.

* More than one response can be given.

Thank you for your time and interest. Please return the questionnaire in the envelope provided.

Figure 6.4 (Continued)

6.6 USING DATA CODING SHEETS

In some research projects, the data may already exist on forms not suitable for keypunching; or for some reason, a suitable form cannot be developed for use as the data are collected. In these instances, the collected data must be transcribed onto data coding sheets to be processed. A data coding sheet is shown in Figure 6.5. Note that it has 80 columns, corresponding to the columns on a computer card. You simply transcribe the data into the appropriate columns, and the data then can be processed easily.

The disadvantages are that transcription takes time and that errors can be made. However, if the data collection form does not exist, a coding sheet is necessary to get the data processed.

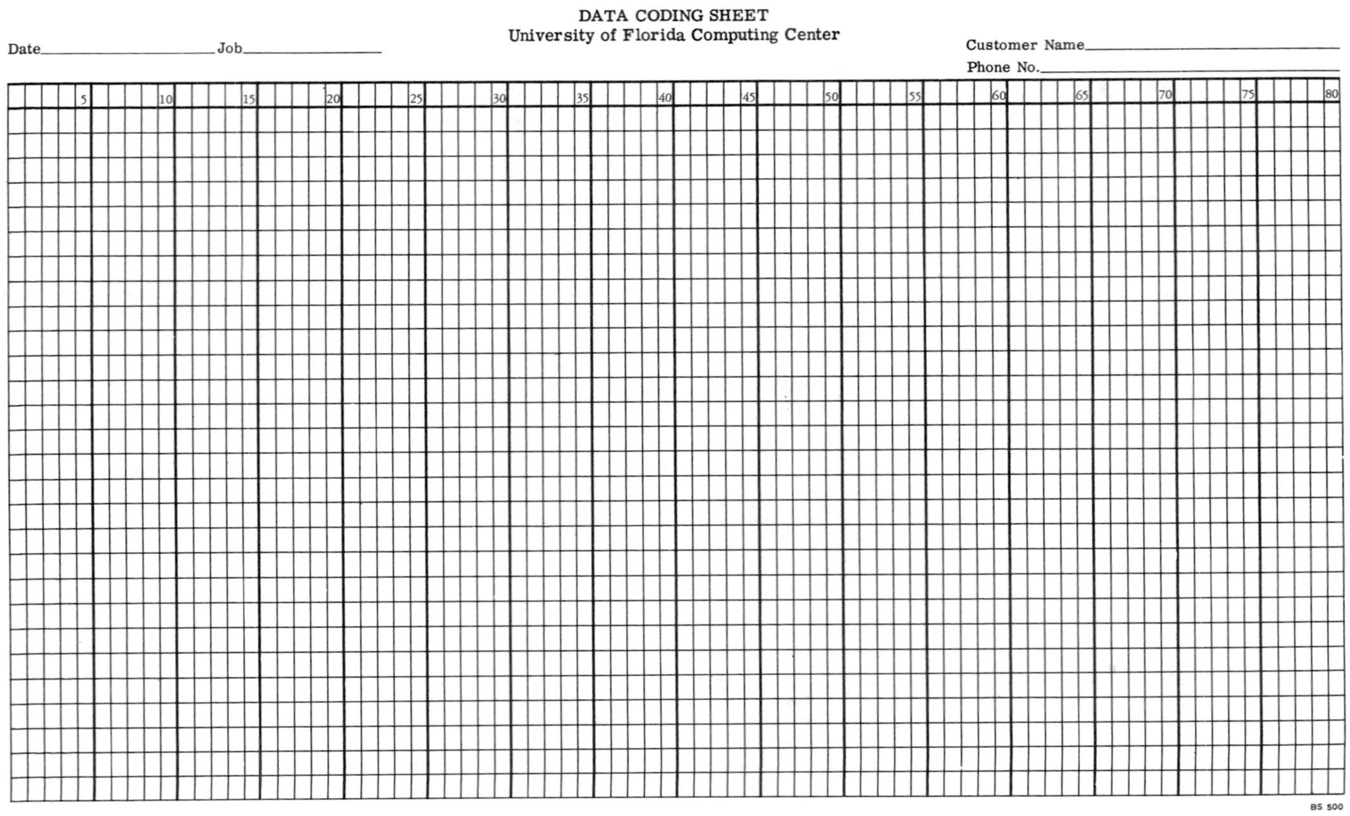

DATA CODING SHEET
University of Florida Computing Center

Date__________ Job__________ Customer Name__________

Phone No.__________

5 10 15 20 25 30 35 40 45 50 55 60 65 70 75 80

BS 500

Figure 6.5 Data coding sheet.

6.7 DESIGNING YOUR DATA COLLECTION FORM

Consider these questions when designing the data collection form for your research project.

6.7.1 All Data Collection Forms

- Have you defined an appropriate identification name or number that is unique for each experimental unit in the project?
- Have you considered all the demographic responses that you wish to obtain?
- Have you decided on all the other responses you wish to measure, including all factors and response variables?
- For each non-numerical response, have you defined appropriate response categories that will cover all possible answers adequately?
- Have you allocated enough columns for the answer to each response?

6.7.2 Questionnaire Forms

Are all questions stated clearly and is answer space laid out clearly so that the respondent understands what you want?

Are all responses coded clearly and are columns for answers marked so that the keypuncher can process the data collection forms accurately and efficiently?

6.8 KEY POINTS

A questionnaire is unique in that it is filled out by many people who usually receive only written instructions regarding how to answer questions. Take particular care to ask only relevant questions to minimize the questionnaire's length. Also, you must review each question with categorical responses to see that all reasonable categories are included. Questions requiring numerical responses should clearly show the number of spaces that should be filled in. Finally, you should differentiate clearly between questions that allow only one response and those that allow multiple responses. Remember that the appearance and clarity of your questionnaire will influence the response rate.

6.9 THE NEXT STEP

The next step in the research design process is to see whether you can and should use a repeated measure or blocking design. This design concept has the double advantage of increasing the information obtained in a study while often reducing its cost. This concept applies only to experimental studies, so if you are planning an observational study, you may proceed to Chapter 7.

REFERENCES

1. Rimm, A. A., Hartz, A. J., Kalbfleisch, J. H., Anderson, A. J., and Hoffmann, R. G. 1980. *Basic biostatistics in medicine and epidemiology*. New York: Appleton-Century-Crofts.
2. Polit, D. F., and Hungler, B. P. 1978. *Nursing research: principles and methods*. New York: Lippincott.

CHAPTER 7

Step Four: Increasing Information and Saving Resources: Repeated Measure and Block Designs

7.1 INTRODUCTION

In any research project, the goal is to *maximize* the amount of information obtained for a *minimum* of time, money, and other resources. Repeated measures and blocking are important concepts in the achievement of this goal. Both concepts require you to have control over assigning the factor levels to the experimental units. Thus, these concepts apply only to experimental studies.

7.2 REPEATED MEASURES

The concept of repeated measures involves measurement of the response variable on the *same* experimental unit under more than one factor level combination. In the biological sciences, each person or animal usually is his or her own control, and the response variable is measured repeatedly under different factor level combinations.

In any experimental study, you should consider using a repeated measure design. To evaluate one, ask yourself two questions:

1. Is it physically possible to use a repeated measure design?
2. If a repeated measure design is possible, will additional information be gained by its use?

7.3 WHAT IS A REPEATED MEASURE DESIGN?

Let us introduce the concept of repeated measure with a simple example.

Project 7.1 Comparison of drugs for response time to a stimulus

The objective of a researcher's project is **to compare Drug A and Drug B to determine whether there is any difference in their ability to affect response time to some stimulus.** The researcher plans to choose a representative group of people and administer one of the drugs to a person. Then the researcher will measure the time that it takes a person to respond to some stimulus. The important terms for this project are

Universe	All people who possibly could receive one of these drugs
Experimental unit	Each individual person
Response variable	Time in seconds to respond to some stimulus. [Note that this response variable *probably* should be considered continuous.]
Population	The collection of response times for each person in the universe
U-sample	The collection of people participating in the study
P-sample	The collection of response times for people included in the study
QUALITATIVE FACTOR	Type of drug
Level 1:	Drug A
Level 2:	Drug B

This factor will be experimental, because the researcher will assign the drugs to the people in the study.

One possible extraneous factor could be age, because young people generally would have faster reaction times than would older people.

This study will be prospective: the researcher will be collecting the response variable measurements at some future time after administration of the drug.

The researcher must now consider whether each experimental unit (person) should receive one level of the factor (Drug A or Drug B) or both levels. Several important considerations affect this decision.

First, the researcher may have to pay people to get their cooperation for this study. Because the total time to participate in the study is only a few minutes, \$5.00 will be offered to each participant for coming in to the researcher's laboratory and participating in the study. If the effect of a drug wears off quickly after the response time to a stimulus is measured, then the researcher should consider administering the second drug to each participant after a reasonable amount of waiting time. The repeated measure design will usually be considered only if the experimental unit can be returned to its baseline, pre-experimental condition. However, in Chapter 11, we introduce a repeated measure design for situations where the experimental unit does not return to its baseline measurement. The result of the repeated measure design in this study is that twice as many response variable measurements are being collected for the same amount of money. Even if the researcher had to pay twice as much to the participant, more information often could be gained with half as many people receiving both drugs.

Next, the researcher must consider how much the response variable normally differs between experimental units. For instance, if the reaction time to a stimulus (response variable) differs from person to person regardless of drug given, there will be a gain in information from exposing each person to each drug. By measuring a person's response time to both drugs, one can make a relative comparison of the two drugs. If only a single response time is measured on an individual for one drug, then a low reading could result from either 1) a drug effect or 2) normally fast reaction time by the experimental unit.

For example, suppose two people enter the study. One person receives Drug A and the other person receives Drug B. Assume that the range of reaction times for all people is from 2 to 10 sec: the fastest possible response time we might see would be 2 sec, while the slowest would be 10 sec. Suppose the resulting measurements on these two people were as shown in Table 7.1. For person 1, we do not know whether 1) this person has a normally fast reaction time or 2) Drug A speeded up the response time. We have a similar concern about the slow response of person 2. If instead we chose only one person for the study and measured his or her reaction time under both drugs, the results might appear as in Table 7.2. We still have the same two readings as in Table 7.1, but now we have the additional information that Drug A reduced response

Table 7.1 Response times of two persons to drugs A and B

	DRUG	
PERSON	*A*	*B*
1	3 sec	
2		8 sec

Table 7.2 Response times of one person to drugs A and B

	DRUG	
PERSON	*A*	*B*
1	3 sec	8 sec

time much more than did Drug B. Therefore, we have gained more information by measuring one person under both drugs than we did from two people, each under one drug. Thus, fewer people would be needed to answer the research objective if a repeated measure design were employed.

In a similar situation where both drugs *cannot* be administered to one person, there are other means of obtaining more information on each experimental unit. One way is to consider each person as his or her own control and to measure response time to the stimulus *before* administering either drug. This method provides a baseline measurement of response time, which then can be compared to the response time measured under Drug A or Drug B. In this particular situation, one can consider the drug factor as having three levels—no drug, Drug A, and Drug B—and each person would receive two levels of this factor. Each person would be measured under the no-drug condition and then under either Drug A and Drug B. A second advantage of using each person as his or her own control is that often this measurement is easily obtained, and therefore valuable information is obtained for little cost.

7.4 QUANTITATIVE AND QUALITATIVE FACTORS IN A REPEATED MEASURE DESIGN

In a repeated measure design, the order of assignment of the factor levels usually is handled differently for a qualitative factor from the way it is for a quantitative factor. If the factor is qualitative, the levels represent different forms of some treatment, and the researcher often can assign the treatments in any order. We shall see in Chapter 11 that the order of assignment of factor levels should not be the same for all experimental units and, in fact, should be properly randomized. A repeated measure design in which the researcher can randomize the order of assignment of the factor levels is called a **changeover** or **crossover design.** Project 7.1, in which we compared two drugs (or two factor levels, in general) is called a two-period changeover (or crossover) design. More details on changeover and crossover designs can be found in references 1 through 3.

The most common quantitative factor studied in a repeated measure design is time. For example, a response variable measurement is obtained on an experimental unit at times 0 (baseline), 15 min, 30 min, 1 h, and 2, 4, 5, 8, 12, and 24 h after some treatment. Obviously, the researcher cannot control the order of assignment of these factor levels. Instead, they occur sequentially and have the same order for all people.

The distinction is very important between a factor, usually qualitative, in which the researcher can decide on the order of assignment of the levels and a factor, usually quantitative, in which the order of assignment is the same for all experimental units and is unalterable. These two designs are analyzed through very different statistical procedures, so the researcher must distinguish between the two types of factors.

7.5 THE CONCEPT OF BLOCKING

Blocking is a very common practice in the agricultural sciences. Assume that a piece of farmland is divided into 10 one-acre plots, each plot representing an experimental unit. If the response variable is yield of corn in bushels, the yield should be similar on all plots if all are fertilized and watered similarly and overall treated in the same way. The 10 plots then would be said to be **homogeneous** and together would form a **block.** Then, if different treatment plans are used on the plots, differences in yield can be attributed to treatment differences.

Blocks on farms in different locations also are assumed to have homogeneous plots within a block, but *between* blocks (or farms), the plots are considered **heterogeneous:** that is, yield of corn may differ between farms.

An analogy to this example in the biomedical sciences is litters of animals. Most response variable measurements vary widely among animals, but a litter of animals might be considered relatively homogeneous on some response variable measurements. Thus, if we wished to compare the effect of four different drugs on some response in rats, and if rats within a litter were considered relatively similar on the response variable in the absence of any drug, we might select four rats from each of a number of litters. The rats should be chosen at random from the litter. (Methods for doing so will be discussed in Chapter 8.) Within each litter, the four rats are assigned to the four drugs in such a way that each drug is given to exactly one rat. The assignment of the rats to the drugs is done through an appropriate randomization scheme to be discussed in Chapter 11. Then, the differences in the response variable can be attributed mainly to the drug, and we can look for a consistent trend over all litters.

This type of blocking is used less often in biomedical research, and you should be very careful about using a block design. The reason is that animals and people differ greatly on most physiological measurements, and even family members are different enough so that the assumption of homogeneity in the block usually is not valid. Thus, while the repeated measure design is very popular in biomedical research, blocking experiments are used less frequently. For more information on block designs, see references 4 through 7.

7.6 THE CONCEPT OF MATCHED PAIRS

In Project 7.1, another means of gaining additional information would be to find pairs of people who are very similar in reaction time and to treat each pair as a block. For example, if age and sex are determined to be the only possible extraneous factors, two 29-year-old males might be chosen to form a block, with one male receiving Drug A and the other, Drug B. Then we would assume that any difference between their response times results from the drugs they received. This arrangement is an example of a **matched pairs design.**

The matched pairs design is used when the possible extraneous factors can be identified and the pool of experimental units for the study is large enough to match on the extraneous factors. The disadvantages of such a design are the need to identify all possible extraneous factors and the need for a large enough pool of experimental units to provide the matched samples. For more information on matched samples, including a comprehensive list of references, see references 8 through 12.

One area where matched pair designs are used frequently is in dentistry. Each side of the mouth often is considered an experimental unit, and two competing treatments can be applied, one to each side. Project 2.1, the study to evaluate two dental sealants, would most likely be done as a matched pair design. If the researcher feels that the side on which a participant chewed could influence the caries rate, which is the response variable, then chewing side should be treated as an extraneous factor and the two sealants should be assigned so that each occurs equally often on the chewing side. Chapter 11 will deal with randomization techniques for balancing over extraneous factors.

Another form of matching is **group matching.** Instead of trying to match individuals, the researcher attempts to match the group members overall on potential extraneous factors. Thus, if age and sex are considered to be extraneous factors, the researcher would strive to obtain a similar proportion of men and women in each factor level and a similar age spread in all factor levels. This type of matching is simpler than matched pairs but, of course, not as exact. Group matching is a reasonable, practical alternative to matched pairs in many studies.

Let us now define formally what is meant by repeated measures and blocking and relate these definitions to two of our examples.

7.7 DEFINITION OF REPEATED MEASURE AND BLOCKING

Complete repeated measure design is used when each experimental unit received *every* factor level combination being studied and has the response variable measured under each combination.

Complete block design is used when experimental units can be grouped homogeneously into a block so that *every* factor level combination occurs an equal number of times in the block and each experimental unit in the block receives exactly one factor level combination.

The factor level combinations in the above definitions refer to studies in which more than one factor is being studied. For example, in Project 3.1, the two factors being studied were

Factor 1:	Type of antidiarrheic drug
Level 1:	Drug A
Level 2:	Drug B
Factor 2:	Nutrition program
Level 1:	None
Level 2:	New program

Each person included in the study will receive one level from each of the factors and then will have the response variable, weight loss, measured. There are four possible factor level combinations in this study. They are

Combination 1	Drug A, no nutrition program
Combination 2	Drug A, new nutrition program
Combination 3	Drug B, no nutrition program
Combination 4	Drug B, new nutrition program

Project 3.1 would be a complete repeated measure design if each experimental unit (person undergoing surgery) could have the response variable (initial weight loss) measured under each factor level combination. In this particular project, the repeated measure design is not readily used, because after receiving one factor level combination and having weight loss measured, the experimental unit cannot be returned to its baseline, pre-experimental condition. Even though a patient's drug and nutrition program can be changed for the second month, weight loss will be less in each month after surgery. This trend leads to an unfair advantage for the factor level combination assigned first.

If the research project has only a single experimental factor to be evaluated, the factor level combinations then are the levels of the single factor.

Incomplete repeated measures or blocking results when, for each experimental unit or block, the response variable is measured under more than one factor level combination but not under all factor level combinations. It is very important to be able to distinguish between complete and incomplete repeated measures or blocking, because the choice of statistical analysis differs for these designs. (For further discussion, see reference 13.)

For Project 7.1, there is only one factor to consider. Therefore, if the two possible levels, Drug A and Drug B, are considered, a complete repeated measure design is used if each person received both drugs. Complete blocking would be used if pairs of "similar" people were selected and one of each pair received Drug A and the other, Drug B. No repeated measure design or blocking is employed if each person's response time is measured under only one drug and there is no pairing or matching of people.

If the situation is considered in which each person serves as his or her own control, our factor now has three levels: no drug, Drug A, and Drug B. A complete repeated measure design occurs if each person's response time is measured under each of the three levels of this factor. Complete blocking occurs if a group of three (or a multiple of three) homogeneous people is selected and each receives one of the three levels of the factor. An incomplete repeated measure design occurs if each person has response time measured under no drug and under either Drug A or Drug B. Incomplete blocking occurs if the block size is greater than one but not a multiple of three. This arrangement may result in the levels of the factor being observed an unequal number of times.

You must decide whether it is possible to use some sort of repeated measures or blocking in a research project. If it is possible, you must decide whether it is *advantageous* to use one.

7.8 WHEN TO USE A REPEATED MEASURE OR BLOCK DESIGN

A main consideration when you are deciding whether or not to use a repeated measure or blocking design is **whether the experimental units provide a wide range of measurements for the response variable in the absence of any factor.** If there is a large difference in the response variable measurements, then it is to your advantage to use one of these designs, because it will increase your information. At the same time, no more time or money may be spent—often, *less* will be expended.

Let us now look at some examples and see whether a repeated measure or blocking design can be used, and if so, whether its use is advantageous.

Project 7.2 Evaluation of the influence of SO_2 on breathing

Refer to Project 4.2, whose objective was **to evaluate the influence on humans either with or without breathing problems of breathing SO_2.** The factors and their levels were

QUALITATIVE FACTORS

Factor 1: Group
Level 1: Normals (no breathing problems)
Level 2: Asthmatics

Factor 2: Breathing what gas?
Level 1: Air only
Level 2: Air and SO_2

Factor 3: Time spent in chamber
Level 1: 0 (baseline measurement)
Level 2: 0.5 h
Level 3: 1 h
Level 4: 2 h
Level 5: 3 h

Can and should a repeated measure or blocking design be employed? There are 20 possible combinations of the three factors, as we determine by multiplying the number of levels of each factor ($2 \times 2 \times 5 = 20$). Each person can have the response variables (vital capacity, FEV_1, MMFR, FRC, and R_{aw}) measured under all combinations of factors 2 and 3 because these factors are both experimental. However, factor 1 is observational, as each person can be in only one of the two groups, and the researcher has no control over the group into which each experimental unit falls. Thus, the study cannot be a complete repeated measure design (because of Factor 1), but it can be an incomplete repeated measure design, because the response variable can be obtained under more than one factor level combination.

We must decide whether we can measure the response variable practically under each combination of factors 2 and 3. Can we measure a person's breathing for three hours while he or she breathes one of the gases listed in factor 2 and then have the participant repeat the experiment for three more hours while breathing the second gas? This approach is advisable only if the participant can return on another day for the second regimen, because he or she should return to baseline, pre-experimental conditions before receiving the second gas.

If the logistics of this problem can be resolved, we must decide whether or not repeated measures will increase our information. To answer this question, we must know something about the response variables under normal breathing conditions. For example, if vital capacity differs widely among people when they are breathing normally, then more information is gained by the use of repeated measures on factor 2. Otherwise, no additional information is gained from repeated measures. Regardless of the experimenter's decision on factor 2, this project is an example of an incomplete repeated measure design, because the response variables will be measured under every level of factor 3.

Project 7.3 Evaluation of factors related to potency retained by a drug

A hospital is considering the use of disposable syringes. A pharmacist in the hospital plans an experiment whose objective is **to evaluate the relationship of type of syringe, storage temperature, length of storage, and amount of drug stored in a syringe on the potency retained of a certain drug in these syringes.** The important terms for this research project are

Universe The total amount of this drug of interest

Experimental unit Each individual syringe of drug

Response variable Percent of potency retained by the drug at the end of the storage period. (Note: the initial potency of the drug is 100 percent.)

Population	The collection of measurements of potency retained by all syringes in the universe if they were stored for an appropriate time
U-sample	The collection of syringes of drug used in the study
P-sample	The collection of potency measurements made on the drugs in the syringes included in the study

Factors

QUALITATIVE FACTOR

Factor 1:	Type of storage syringe
Level 1:	Glass
Level 2 :	Plastic

QUANTITATIVE FACTORS

Factor 2:	Storage temperature
Level 1:	40°F (refrigerated)
Level 2:	70°F (room temperature)
Factor 3:	Time stored
Level 1:	30 days
Level 2:	60 days
Level 3:	90 days
Factor 4:	Amount of drug stored
Level 1:	40 mg
Level 2:	30 mg
Level 3:	20 mg
Level 4:	10 mg

Each of the factors under study is experimental, because the researcher will have complete control over assigning the levels of each factor to the experimental units. One large batch of the drug will be divided into individual syringes for this study, so there should be no extraneous factors. Also, this study will be prospective, because the data will be collected in the future after the project is designed.

In this project, the response variable measurement will be a number between 0 percent and 100 percent and should be considered continuous.

Because the experimental units all come from the same batch of drug, there is no difference among them, so the concepts of repeated measures and blocking do not seem to be important in this study. If multiple batches were used, each batch could be considered a block. The syringes of drug within a batch should be homogeneous, but the various batches could differ. Also, it would be difficult to use repeated measures on factor 1, because an experimental unit cannot be stored in both a plastic and a glass syringe. If it were stored in a plastic syringe for a while, the potency retained could be measured, but then the experimental unit could not be returned to its pre-experimental condition, because some potency will be lost. Thus, the same experimental unit cannot be measured similarly in a glass syringe, and repeated measures is not advised. Similar problems prohibit the use of repeated measures on factors 2 and 4. For factor 3, repeated measures are possible but may not be advisable. The same syringe can have potency measured at 30, 60, and 90 days, but the researcher might worry that the drug would become contaminated when it was removed from its syringe for potency measurement during the experiment.

A repeated measure design thus is probably not necessary or advisable, and blocking would be considered only if multiple batches of the drug were used in the study.

Project 7.4 Evaluation of a new drug to treat epilepsy

Refer to Project 4.5, whose objective is **to evaluate the relationship between type of drug administered (Drug X and Drug Y) and the monthly epileptic seizure rate of mentally retarded people.** An experimental unit in this study is an individual mentally retarded person, and the response variable is the monthly epileptic seizure rate. In Project 4.5, the researcher decided that each person would have to be followed for at least three months under a factor level to establish the seizure rate effectively, because the occurrence of seizures would vary from month to month.

A crossover design is possible since the response variable can be measured before the participant begins using Drug X (while on Drug Y, or in a control condition) and again after use of Drug X. Since the monthly seizure rate probably is quite different for the individual participants in the study regardless of drug given, a crossover design probably will increase information. Therefore, the researcher should try to incorporate it into the design of the project.

The researcher might reject a crossover design in this study for only one reason: it will require the project to run for a longer time. If half the people in the study are switched immediately to Drug X, a one-month washout period is used to allow all effects of Drug Y to clear the body, and then each person in the two groups is followed for three months, the study can be completed in four months. If a baseline (or Drug Y) seizure rate is obtained on everyone for three months before everyone is switched to Drug X, and then the seizure rate is obtained again for three months after a one-month washout period, the study would require seven months for completion.

If the available U-sample is small, the crossover design will be the only alternative that might yield enough information to answer the research objective. Thus, if the researcher cannot afford to carry out this study for seven months and the available U-sample is too small to yield conclusive results under the alternative design for only four months, the project should be restructured or dropped.

Project 7.5 Evaluation of educational procedures to reduce prejudice of grade school children

Refer to Project 4.3, which had as its objective **to evaluate a newly developed educational procedure to determine whether the attitude of grade school children who are prejudiced toward handicapped children is improved.** The experimental units in this study are the children prejudiced toward the handicapped, and the factor of interest is type of educational procedure used to eliminate prejudice.

Since the children have a measure of prejudice determined before any educational experience, the response variable is measured under Level 1 (no education). All children can experience the newly developed educational procedure (Level 2) and then have their prejudice measured a second time. Therefore, the researcher would be using complete repeated measures on the experimental units. However, an additional effect is present in this project that may influence the results. The presence of the researcher in the classroom may have an effect on the prejudice of some students, regardless of whether or not they receive the new educational procedure. This effect must be measured through the use of a control group. Consider the following three levels for the factor of interest.

Level 1: Baseline prejudice before the researcher begins the project

Level 2: No educational procedure, but researcher present in classroom

Level 3: Researcher present and educational procedure presented

Under this plan, all students are measured under Level 1. Then the students are divided into two groups. Group 1 receives Level 2, while Group 2 receives Level 3. Group 1 is the control group and measures the influence of the researcher in the classroom. The influence of the educational procedure now can be evaluated and compared to no education. This design is an example of incomplete repeated measures, because each experimental unit is subjected to two of the three possible levels of the factor in this study.

7.9 REPEATED MEASURES OR BLOCKING IN YOUR RESEARCH PROJECT

For the project whose objective you listed in Chapter 2, you should evaluate the effect of repeated measures or blocking on the experimental units. The experimental units and factor for your research project were defined in Chapter 2, so you now are ready to answer the following questions.

- Is either the method of repeated measures, blocking, or matching physically possible for this research project?
- If the method of repeated measures or blocking is possible, will additional information be gained? (Or, is there a basic difference in the response variable between experimental units in the absence of any factor?)

- If the method of repeated measures or blocking is employed, is it complete or incomplete? Be sure to evaluate each factor level combination to be studied.

7.10 KEY POINTS

This chapter discussed two important concepts to consider when you are designing an experiment. The big advantages of repeated measures and blocking is that they can *increase* the amount of information obtained in a study without an increase in cost. If you are submitting a grant proposal, you should be especially concerned about designing the most efficient study possible and showing the funding agency that you are maximizing the amount of information that can be obtained in the study.

These concepts are complex and hence are often overlooked or misused, but they are important.

7.11 THE NEXT STEP

We are now at the point of considering the experimental units to include in the study, or how we shall take the U-sample. You should consider taking some type of probability sample that will, we hope, result in a group of experimental units that are representative of the entire universe. Unfortunately, in most biomedical research projects a probability sample is not practical or even possible and, in this case, you must try to determine how the U-sample may differ from the entire universe and how this difference may influence the conclusions that are drawn.

REFERENCES

1. Hills, M., and Armitage, P. 1979. The two-period cross-over clinical trial. *British Journal of Clinical Pharmacology* 8: 7–20.
2. Cochran, W. G., and Cox, G. M. 1957. *Experimental designs.* London: Wiley.
3. Rimm, A. A., Hartz, A. J., Kalbfleisch, J. H., Anderson, A. J., and Hoffmann, R. G. 1980. *Basic biostatistics in medicine and epidemiology.* New York: Appleton-Century-Crofts.
4. Mendenhall, W. 1968. *Introduction to linear models and the design and analysis of experiments.* Belmont, Calif.: Wadsworth.
5. Ott, L. 1977. *An introduction to statistical methods and data analysis.* North Scituate, Mass.: Duxbury.
6. Kleinbaum, D. G., and Kupper, L. L. 1978. *Applied regression analysis and other multivariable methods.* North Scituate, Mass.: Duxbury.

7. Steel, R. G. D., and Torrie, J. H. 1960. *Principles and procedures of statistics.* New York: McGraw-Hill. Pp. 132, 133.

8. Feinstein, A. R. 1977. *Clinical biostatistics.* St. Louis: Mosby. Pp. 56, 193, 202.

9. Feinstein, A. R. 1970. Clinical biostatistics V: The architecture of clinical research (concluded). *Clin. Pharmacol. Ther.* 11: 757.

10. Feinstein, A. R. 1973. Clinical biostatistics XIX: Ambiguity and abuse in the twelve different concepts of "Control." *Clin. Pharmacol. Ther.* 14:119.

11. Feinstein, A. R. 1973. Clinical biostatistics XX: The epidemiologic trohoc, the ablative risk ratio and "Retrospective Research." *Clin. Pharmacol. Ther.* 14: 296.

12. Colton, T. 1974. *Statistics in medicine.* Boston: Little, Brown.

13. Marks, R. 1982. *Analyzing research data.* Belmont, Calif.: Lifetime Learning Publications.

CHAPTER 8

Step Five: Choosing the Participants for the Study

8.1 INTRODUCTION

As we pointed out in Chapter 2, the objective of any research project is to make some decision about a universe and the factors to which it is exposed. To arrive at this decision, we collect response variable measurements on a group of experimental units, and we then extrapolate the results of the analysis to the entire population of response variable measurements. We then interpret these results as they relate to the universe being observed. If the conclusion is to be valid, the group of experimental units selected must represent the entire universe. Thus, it is important to know how to choose a representative group of experimental units from the universe and to understand what will happen if a nonrepresentative sample is chosen. A **bias** exists when the levels of an extraneous factor occur disproportionately in the U-sample. For example, if the universe of interest were all adults and 90% of the U-sample were women, sex would create a bias in the study. Thus, you must be able to identify potential biases and control for them by the proper selection of the U-sample.

Although often it is not possible, you should try to use a probability sampling scheme. The four most common probability sampling schemes are 1) simple random sampling, 2) stratified sampling, 3) cluster sampling, and 4) systematic sampling. The different types of sampling schemes have advantages in different research situations.

This chapter discusses each of these four types of sampling schemes and when each should be used. It also discusses the problems that arise when we draw inferences about a population where a representative sample cannot be chosen. You must understand the limitations on the conclusions drawn under these conditions.

8.2 THE IMPORTANCE OF A REPRESENTATIVE SAMPLE

If a political pollster had predicted that Jimmy Carter would defeat Ronald Reagan by a landslide in the 1980 presidential election and had based these conclusions on a random sample of voters polled in Plains, Georgia, few people would have expressed much confidence in that prediction. The reason is that although the people polled may have been representative of the voters in Plains, Georgia, they hardly were representative of the entire voting universe of the United States. The result of this biased geographical sampling would have led to an erroneous conclusion.

Similarly, a single litter of beagles in a research project may be representative of the beagles available from a particular animal resource center, but it may not be representative of all beagles. Some characteristics present in these beagles may be genetic and may not be present in other beagles. A project that involves these beagles might reach an erroneous conclusion.

Occasionally, two independent researchers perform identical research projects and arrive at different conclusions. One major cause of this discrepancy is that the experimental units were chosen in different manners and were not both representative of the same universe.

In many biomedical research projects, truly representative samples cannot be selected from the universes of interest. When the experimental units are to be drawn from hospital patients or outpatient clinics, you are limited to those people who happen to appear on the scene at the time when the sample is chosen. The fact that a representative sample cannot be chosen does not invalidate the research or serve as an unfair criticism of your work. However, you must realize that the inferences drawn may have some limitations, and you should try to identify the potential biases that may be introduced to the response variable because of the lack of complete representation.

Some biases, such as sex, age, race, and height, can be controlled easily in many studies by the proper inclusion of experimental units in the study. You can determine the number of males and females to include in the study and achieve those numbers. Similarly, you can determine the desirable age frequencies for the study and often can choose the U-sample to satisfy the age requirements.

In some research projects, only a few experimental units may be available, and you include all of them in the study. For example, suppose the universe of interest is all people who have had gastric partition surgery. A hospital may perform only a few of these operations in a month, or possibly in a year. You then would include in the project any person coming to the hospital for this operation during the time of the research project. In this situation, you must be especially careful to realize the possible shortcomings of such a sampling scheme. The sample probably will come from a small geographical region and will include only patients having this surgery in one hospital. Also, if the patients are collected over a short period of time, any current epidemics or illnesses may bias the sample. Of course, if sampling every possible patient is the only available sampling scheme, you must use it. The important thing is to try to choose as representative as possible a sample from the universe.

Even if you feel that a representative U-sample has been drawn from the local geographic region, a geographical bias is very common. This bias occurs when physiological differences exist between geographic locations, and hence, the response variable measurements differ between locations. Geographical bias cannot be controlled unless this U-sample can be chosen from various geographical regions, and because this approach usually is impossible, geographical bias often is present. This is one of the reasons why two independent researchers, performing similar studies in different parts of the country, may arrive at different conclusions.

Another type of bias, called **Berkson's bias,** was pointed out by Joseph Berkson in 1946 (reference 1), and an example of this bias was pointed out later (reference 2). Suppose you were interested in women using birth control pills and in determining the incidence of some disease, such as cervical cancer. You compare women using the pill to those not using the pill and find that, indeed, the incidence of the disease is much higher in the group using the pill. Can you conclude that the pill is a cause of this disease? Probably not, at least not without much more evidence to substantiate this conclusion. One possible explanation for this result is that women using the pill receive more medical examinations than do members of the other group and hence face a higher detection rate, even if the incidence rate is no higher. This phenomenon was pointed out by Berkson, and it must be carefully considered in all studies. Thus, in addition to being similar on all basic demographic factors, the groups should be similar in their medical treatments and health care opportunities. In general, the choice of a control or comparison group is very important. You must make sure that it is similar to the experimental group in all important aspects.

The point to remember is that when you deal with human subjects, it often is difficult to choose a representative sample from the universe of interest. You must be careful to identify potential biases in the chosen sample. More information on this topic can be found in references 3 through 9.

Let us now examine the four different types of sampling schemes.

8.3 SIMPLE RANDOM SAMPLING

Simple random sampling is the most commonly used of the four sampling procedures in biomedical research projects. A formal definition of simple random sampling is as follows:

> If a U-sample of size n is drawn from a universe of size N in such a way that every possible U-sample of size n has the same chance of being selected, that sampling procedure is called **simple random sampling.**

A simple random sample can be chosen if the experimental units in the universe are numbered from 1 to N. The experimental units included in the study are determined by the numbers chosen from a random number table such as Table 8.1. Pick any starting point in the table and move through the table in any pattern to choose the numbers of the experimental units to include in the study. If the size of the universe is $N = 7800$, omit selected numbers greater than that. As an example, if we decide to select 10 numbers randomly, we choose a starting point at random (throw a dart or pick a point with our eyes closed). Starting at line 11 and row 5 and using only the last 4 digits of each number, we choose numbers by moving down column 5, using numbers in odd rows. The U-sample then would include experimental units with the following numbers:

6859	4207	1349
3213	4389	3483
5631	349	
7375	5151	

Note that 8683 and 9706 were skipped because no experimental units would have those numbers. Also, if any number is repeated, its second occurrence is deleted because each experimental unit is included only one time.

This method also could be used to select charts in medical records.

It often is impossible to select a true random sample because the experimental units in a universe either are uncountable or are unknown until they present themselves to the researcher. For example, the universe of all adult Americans is uncountable for sampling purposes. Likewise, the universe of all people facing gastric partition surgery cannot be identified, and experimental units are identified only when they are referred to the surgical department. In these situations, random sampling cannot be used, but we still should try to choose the U-sample so that it is as representative as possible of the entire universe. We also should try to identify any potential biases and determine how they may influence or limit the results of the study. For more information on taking random samples, see references 10 through 12.

Table 8.1 Part of a random number table

Row/Cols.	*1*	*2*	*3*	*4*	*5*	*6*	*7*	*8*
1	23184	01486	25898	33892	08491	63986	21256	86789
2	11685	04099	92644	76810	48735	98662	25055	04807
3	06144	65195	46601	34820	24358	87556	54102	96090
4	98364	20450	13760	67618	69880	84749	78351	48472
5	69537	12795	54410	78098	09070	43721	19420	06641
6	23506	68756	88999	15247	63350	26544	34086	86382
7	36773	48452	48130	24144	01800	53886	64278	24573
8	08496	95598	22561	95965	91155	55006	87084	29184
9	10488	87500	13209	17977	45809	17758	64748	29281
10	37221	85058	81146	23542	77809	38590	94670	25022
11	55820	82768	97598	42116	46859	72544	59406	37660
12	56069	58719	93951	49247	10322	83255	76668	59540
13	00406	24591	11746	16580	73213	92952	49324	04103
14	73926	75662	52678	51851	38206	32457	15401	55883
15	34380	40800	28601	98890	55631	91188	98079	20507
16	62178	32469	11524	87622	73473	67153	55695	74695
17	10382	96726	83613	84065	87375	16959	31743	16264
18	54713	63222	87189	90330	90635	05801	04873	14121
19	43547	95202	74731	04624	24207	57472	38892	58270
20	47916	39504	58872	71245	26703	04357	32760	09806
21	11511	76561	62404	30587	84389	37435	70598	50919
22	00676	70397	68273	69136	81189	56278	71680	34893
23	54412	18633	69582	69473	48683	19053	40437	36106
24	34378	02482	19590	60273	16105	92521	16457	00028
25	74887	36751	81713	66303	60349	02036	24483	93225
26	32910	19841	79523	58425	55963	81544	24415	53355
27	38072	83747	46748	03595	25151	23589	61310	39170
28	42657	44057	77272	14862	87774	29304	15379	80518
29	71604	49953	75135	01369	11349	58419	51991	28337
30	72507	34212	04534	18353	61050	79256	71672	04662
31	65619	63202	39823	17144	49706	18733	60103	52620
32	93847	86887	15511	95167	87803	12360	38120	86432
33	72754	88824	76262	45941	33483	54240	11717	41413
34	40562	36165	26900	09076	42544	47070	22045	23972
35	08147	29653	82401	20278	18441	52144	95410	61611
36	09041	53627	17900	61347	62285	39346	93273	52927
37	49433	26020	18689	10175	22843	37154	62254	17609
38	58159	48356	30213	90750	46539	82643	84128	46441
39	36749	55757	08075	23152	27451	71477	25825	51300
40	09333	66934	68035	73556	57315	07918	89433	15158
41	72733	34196	36009	04228	75525	54820	62196	42080
42	46420	93443	98067	23532	19127	83629	56514	07224
43	22521	14169	50439	35923	72828	24389	09942	06843
44	15817	49464	49508	91950	18987	15733	35194	08283
45	13749	86009	61815	38257	87621	54892	70137	99983
46	26411	94080	14057	67579	06404	47687	77797	41478
47	36554	77547	43087	68748	50666	58535	06355	13396
48	49587	23873	45914	76687	93393	60447	39148	67456
49	43574	54116	29703	22416	55226	85026	44670	76475
50	19234	72925	61776	83046	54463	72471	26571	84360
51	49944	18547	19612	31781	57060	21572	73657	56115
52	31737	12818	40845	87923	26628	39716	09890	27835
53	33302	11172	73265	66863	74432	92880	44389	56711
54	45983	52634	24818	30089	09398	55638	21429	71025
55	33784	09824	13609	35181	88103	61157	70442	20157
56	83360	38955	17896	85813	64785	51196	56013	24576
57	54026	29834	26095	81754	41335	26109	27888	25848
58	27753	55862	86777	68865	17302	94845	70966	36631
59	59157	24035	58671	89102	39889	24945	55303	90678
60	25550	24939	60661	30514	53959	92543	86112	92834
61	76841	82758	21787	77244	52027	32370	53761	69041
62	85637	05267	31246	59530	24268	87748	83775	16332
63	97187	33836	88391	03701	08511	60593	86836	52833
64	79401	93428	52732	82182	40242	61415	08780	67767
65	72841	42600	93934	63491	02603	59319	80601	71448
66	40728	23504	41819	62240	76392	32002	68450	45285
67	18939	11884	36365	89134	90064	15756	23632	91781
68	66006	67077	77705	00973	69730	55466	32610	84531
69	13118	82017	76132	50650	89156	54612	67002	18225
70	14121	33230	02090	37152	19767	25265	33584	58647
71	95515	30834	36184	55559	80641	38092	24287	92676
72	06459	68544	19173	47045	88515	72354	66197	78281
73	68767	73665	01972	48878	07780	65905	71559	94527
74	26908	57100	95653	44421	00485	65192	87772	91574
75	98010	63343	21444	13130	76335	75257	47393	40674

Table 8.1 (Continued)

Row/Cols.	*1*	*2*	*3*	*4*	*5*	*6*	*7*	*8*
76	21855	20483	60729	80552	42691	09735	18134	84173
77	10881	90200	05049	68331	54558	40855	52864	85512
78	00185	17772	06101	44205	64642	49440	39607	79222
79	97517	82068	25737	72004	73241	74906	51545	20933
80	33286	45551	85967	61651	78352	65264	97015	37366
81	10555	04279	18957	19166	25615	27117	69511	76334
82	55044	37901	17028	96659	58331	75664	97682	56748
83	65131	59664	82658	42337	67453	84696	95336	18609
84	61847	66405	78482	50499	41591	36598	11434	73013
85	38881	88556	77289	11537	17015	72349	80094	52151
86	12580	40144	12028	61940	27645	41522	70593	59306
87	71944	68788	25800	34286	55063	52284	37360	18856
88	28631	05701	21866	07251	78504	21394	69984	26272
89	66955	15690	13640	55603	24860	24206	43208	98119
90	93886	47157	74695	00203	18679	44669	66931	22055
91	89051	82096	88758	58007	32166	25324	36211	06833
92	54732	86095	99713	92064	35182	17307	81259	32299
93	65868	58336	61602	61518	45244	30345	17445	99394
94	20056	81596	88622	71605	77526	82762	95292	80150
95	87545	72244	05124	23656	94856	51475	50482	67695
96	61244	30243	95618	65095	57721	21994	53854	26251
97	06716	89150	54771	39440	74263	38422	61399	41132
98	12183	66117	37403	36303	50279	53457	64268	68747
99	38520	11888	08492	41389	39226	78392	38768	86598
100	69260	60801	93174	86499	92213	33110	96361	43283
101	60592	80789	26738	99524	08008	96092	33665	08489
102	91362	23377	04632	54452	83034	54410	82455	23003
103	13070	73685	32457	21363	61370	53731	59662	48699
104	99875	00426	75975	16432	84753	48314	17374	18551
105	98590	05908	11099	51927	42574	51014	92835	86623
106	78686	76032	73902	86209	21882	83278	58444	78073
107	82288	30291	10613	73734	57382	25148	71758	39154
108	74181	71775	27614	15052	81434	65260	25488	87213
109	91803	37165	41447	06805	74055	50841	97504	50688
110	95248	46738	28808	91730	12919	37716	00831	69115
111	17269	54362	76551	08658	23355	40300	33649	43119
112	13274	97502	31685	42513	28350	81604	29296	84423
113	11325	47215	51375	74314	98544	43232	06266	15842
114	62144	58151	52944	31171	02238	15381	18208	31283
115	89106	18555	63868	36291	55384	46843	03929	45751
116	38245	00266	71783	58973	71594	95004	37391	45339
117	28250	08715	74478	64610	12136	75842	77713	37240
118	00466	32928	29902	64689	35932	13929	19170	99736
119	68893	95526	06156	66790	49562	92434	41193	32205
120	70191	02720	31500	24588	57262	03115	58368	05117
121	13672	94320	44349	87850	10923	96327	70441	10039
122	31308	93725	43276	52440	60095	31017	12310	09628
123	27724	57930	37009	10311	01982	24728	04033	87637
124	30203	27523	94430	99513	31445	03593	00821	98913
125	38684	76687	94582	54191	91000	52343	43042	19395
126	75763	63198	76661	54579	20822	64300	06223	96116
127	36691	78425	90020	77010	08739	91381	51044	97205
128	39376	97331	44168	43906	40238	94096	73342	61883
129	74381	28473	58771	73787	48461	91548	54111	50464
130	54927	64003	13650	31264	64206	11436	09501	94357
131	66890	29666	98784	77043	65927	40051	40819	46065
132	18803	34798	64307	17922	29735	72278	84526	29183
133	91855	22334	70509	56796	79399	61597	62241	88403
134	89892	18797	37837	42651	36340	70079	30739	39506
135	89414	84309	96895	20567	69638	18393	31952	19372
136	89579	62583	38441	81718	46030	35797	42966	35970
137	62202	30925	63391	13374	79907	10146	26025	18367
138	01752	50236	32816	48895	83318	37887	78530	66720
139	75356	15012	17945	17737	15967	74063	83036	02283
140	72797	03340	50163	95450	35216	82308	57256	17400
141	56513	26903	71009	53676	46081	84851	04059	25513
142	11601	80977	82180	10153	51235	12516	61469	11155
143	95810	94430	95530	78711	01008	54718	52667	79954
144	89550	79727	83067	19274	43387	09468	35991	08630
145	45884	82925	26958	87860	74012	33370	54935	94998
146	40532	33674	69523	86582	86183	91621	88148	07968
147	21871	95220	63242	13644	20854	08014	99436	37541
148	60933	14399	20748	13346	16636	14933	87763	44814
149	01408	71646	64831	26081	59796	03357	37247	11977
150	09640	30985	78439	38337	34257	72860	67162	92314

You must realize that simple random sampling will not guarantee a representative sample of experimental units from the universe, especially in the presence of extraneous factors. Stratified random sampling will provide more information than will simple random sampling when extraneous factors are present.

8.4 STRATIFIED RANDOM SAMPLING

Extraneous factors were introduced in Chapter 2, and examples have been presented throughout this text. An extraneous factor is one that is of no real interest but for which, nonetheless, the response variable measurements may differ for each level. Therefore, we must be assured that there is not a disproportionate number of experimental units at one level of that factor. Stratified random sampling involves selecting a proportionate share of experimental units from each level of the extraneous factor. Each such level is called a **stratum.** As an example, if you are measuring the glucose of adults, this response variable is greater for men than for women. Thus, if a simple random sample is chosen, it is possible to choose a disproportionate number of men or women in the study. Although sex is not of interest to the researcher, it is important to include representative numbers of both men and women in the study. We can achieve this aim through stratified random sampling by considering the two strata of men and women (levels of the extraneous factor) and choosing a random sample from each stratum.

You will recall that the goal in designing a research project is to maximize the amount of information that one can obtain for a minimum of resources expended. For a given sample size, stratified random sampling will provide more information than will simple random sampling by controlling for the extraneous factors. Therefore, stratified random sampling generally is used instead of simple random sampling when extraneous factors are present, and it usually increases the amount of information that can be obtained in a research project. For more information on stratified sampling, see references 10 through 12.

Another type of sampling can reduce the cost of obtaining a response variable in a high-cost project. This type of scheme is called cluster sampling.

8.5 CLUSTER SAMPLING

Suppose Blue Cross would like to examine the medical charts of patients who have filed claims with them in the past year. The purpose is to determine whether the hospital actually performed all the services for which the patient was billed. Assume that Blue Cross has a list of all people who have filed for payment in the past year and that a random sample of patients can be selected from this list with the use of a random number table. Then the person or persons responsible for examining the charts would have to travel all over the country to locate the experimental units or their medical records at their hospitals. This effort would involve a great cost to Blue Cross to measure a response variable on each experimental unit. After meeting the expense of traveling to a hospital to locate a particular medical record, a researcher could survey many medical records at low cost. Therefore, the sampling scheme should allow the researcher to sample more than one medical record in each hospital. Thus, instead of a random sample of hospital patients, a random sample of hospitals throughout the country will first be chosen. Then all the medical records, or a random sample, in the selected hospital will be chosen. This group will not be a true random sample of all medical records in the country, but the increased number of medical records studied makes up for the lack of total randomness in the sample.

In some examples, as in the one presented above, there may be no complete listing of all experimental units. In this situation, it is impossible to choose a simple random sample of medical records, and cluster sampling is an alternative means of choosing a sample.

In general, cluster sampling should be used in two types of situations: 1) when the experimental units tend to occur in clusters and the expense of traveling between clusters is great, and 2) when a listing of all experimental units in the universe is not available. The effect of cluster sampling is to reduce the cost of measuring the response variable on an experimental unit. For more information on cluster sampling, see references 10 through 12.

The fourth and final type of sampling scheme to be discussed is systematic sampling.

8.6 SYSTEMATIC SAMPLING

Systematic sampling can be used when a complete list of all experimental units in the universe is available. This sampling scheme involves selecting at random an experimental unit from the first k experimental units in the listing. Then every kth experimental unit after that in the listing is selected. Systematic sampling has two advantages over simple random sampling in certain sampling situations. One advantage is that systematic sampling is simpler to perform than is simple random sampling, and hence, fewer errors are made in sample selection. Also, the actual process requires less work than does simple random sampling. The second reason is that systematic sampling often provides a more representative sample of the universe than does simple random sampling, in that it is similar to stratified sampling if the list is in some particular order.

As an example, consider the universe of all doctors licensed to practice medicine in a particular state. Assume that the state medical association maintains a list of these doctors by year of graduation. A simple random sample of doctors from this list might yield a majority from the late 1970s or from the early 1950s. If we are interested in a cross sample from all years, a systematic sample will assure that we get it. If the list of experimental units is in any particular order, systematic sampling will guarantee a cross section of experimental units based on their order. If the list is alphabetical, for example, then systematic sampling should be equivalent to simple random sampling, but it still is useful because it is easier to perform.

Systematic sampling also can be used when the experimental units arrive in some order, such as in an outpatient clinic. If every person cannot be included in the study, we may decide to include every fifth or tenth person who comes into the clinic. This systematic sampling should be equivalent to random sampling if the people are arriving in a random fashion.

Excellent references for systematic sampling are available (references 10 through 12).

8.7 AN EXAMPLE USING ALL SAMPLING SCHEMES

Let us look at an example that demonstrates each of the four types of sampling schemes. This example involves "multistage" sampling, because more than one sample is chosen. We shall not go into details about sampling at various stages, because many books on sampling discuss this topic. For more information, see references 5 through 11.

Our example is Project 3.2, which had as its objective **to estimate the rate of generic substitution for all prescriptions filled in the state of Florida for a particular month.**

An experimental unit in this study was a prescription that was filled during the appropriate month. The response variable was simply *yes* or *no*, to denote whether or not a generic substitution was made for that prescription.

The researcher felt that the rate of substitution might differ in various parts of the state. For example, a highly urbanized area such as Miami, with an above-average cost of living, might have a different substitution rate from that in a more rural area with a lower cost of living, such as the Florida panhandle. Thus, although geographic location was not of interest in this study, it was an extraneous factor, and stratified random sampling was the method of choice to control for this factor. Since the state of Florida is divided into six geographic regions by the state pharmacy association, it was decided to take a random sample of pharmacies from each region to insure a cross sample of the entire state. This approach would be stratified sampling with six geographic strata.

Furthermore, the researcher placed all state pharmacies into three groups:

1. independent pharmacies
2. small chains—no more than 10 pharmacies
3. large chains—more than 10 pharmacies

The substitution rate might differ in the three groups, so this grouping was another extraneous factor. Thus, stratified random sampling was used on this factor within each of the six geographic regions.

Because of high travel and per diem expense, the researcher wanted to minimize the number of pharmacies visited and maximize the number of prescriptions sampled at each pharmacy. Thus, instead of sampling prescriptions (which would be virtually impossible, anyhow), the researcher decided to choose pharmacies randomly and then to spend an entire day sampling prescriptions in a pharmacy. This approach is an example of cluster sampling of prescriptions. The researcher now only needed to decide how to select the prescriptions within each pharmacy.

The researcher decided that about 500 prescriptions could be sampled in a day and that samples should be selected to cover the entire month of interest. Because the prescriptions were filed in chronological order, the researcher used systematic sampling to select the prescriptions for the sample. If a pharmacy filled a total of 2000 prescriptions during the month, one of the first four prescriptions on file was selected at random, and then every fourth prescription after that one was selected. If a pharmacy filled 5000 prescriptions one of the first 10 prescriptions was selected at random, and every tenth prescription after that one was selected. Each situation should yield about 500 prescriptions in the sample.

This example illustrates the use of the four types of sampling schemes that are most commonly employed in medical research. The response variable measurements in this project should be the most representative sample one could obtain and also should provide as much information as possible, given the time and travel limitations.

Nothing was mentioned in this example about how many pharmacies to sample. Many sampling books describe what to consider when you are deciding on the sample size (references 10 through 13). The next chapter also will deal with this topic.

8.8 SPECIAL SAMPLING PROBLEMS: VOLUNTEER AND QUESTIONNAIRE SAMPLES

There are two other types of sampling schemes, which share a common problem. They are the "volunteer" sample and the "questionnaire" sample. We obtain the volunteer sample by having people volunteer to participate in the project. An example of this type of sample might be Project 3.3, whose objective is to evaluate the effect of prolonged breathing of SO_2. Two groups, normals and asthmatics, are to be included in the study. The asthmatic group might be selected from a clinic. To obtain the normal group, we might advertise in the local media for heavy smokers to volunteer for a research study.

A questionnaire sample is the returned response to a mailed questionnaire.

The problem with both of these samples is that they may be biased, and it is difficult to identify what type of bias is present. Let us take a look at an example of each kind and try to evaluate the types of bias that may be present.

Refer to Project 3.4, which was a clinical trial experiment to evaluate the flavor and acceptance of a new toothpaste. We must recruit 1000 subjects to use either the new toothpaste or a current commercial brand for 90 days. The subjects will be recruited by advertisement in a local newspaper and radio station. Do you believe that the sample obtained in this manner is representative of all people? First, the sample is restricted to people reading the local paper or listening to that radio station. If the radio station plays rock music, the sample may contain more young people than it should. Another possible bias is that poorer people may tend to volunteer, because they will receive free dental products and a free dental examination at the end of the study. The dental school is located in a college town, and the sample may contain a disproportionate number of college students. Also, housewives with children and working people may find it inconvenient to participate, because the clinic hours are from 9:00 a.m. to 4:00 p.m. Some potential sources of bias can be evaluated (such as age), and others would be difficult to evaluate (such as whether poorer people tend to volunteer). We must be careful in extrapolating the results to the entire universe of people, because some unidentified forms of bias may be present in the sample.

Questionnaire samples suffer from a similar problem. Suppose a nurse wishes to determine the attitude of nurses in one state toward abortion. A list of all nurses is available from the state nursing association and, thus, a random sample of all nurses can be chosen to receive the questionnaire concerning attitude toward abortion. The problem here is that not all the questionnaires will be returned, and the researcher will not know why. Did the nonrespondents lose their questionnaires before returning them? If so, the response is made up of the more organized nurses, and their attitude may be different from that of less organized nurses. Or did some nurses not respond because of lack of interest in the topic? If abortions are illegal, the nurses favoring a change in the law (pro abortion) may be more vocal and may respond to the questionnaire, while nurses with the anti-abortion attitude may tend to be complacent because the law is on their side. The researcher does not know what form of bias, if any, is present in the returned sample.

If you are planning to use a mail-out questionnaire as your method of obtaining data, you should realize that not all people who receive your questionnaire will fill it out and return it. Most researchers are overly optimistic about the return rate they expect for their questionnaires and then become disappointed when only 30% of the questionnaires are returned. You must realize that others will not be as interested in your project as you are, and hence, you must work hard to get them to return your questionnaire. It is important to try to maximize the response rate to your questionnaire as a means of minimizing biases. There are several ways to improve the response rate of a questionnaire. Realize that, even by following this advice on maximizing your response rate, you will not achieve a 100% return. In many studies, an 80% response is about as high as you can hope for realistically.

8.9 MAXIMIZING RESPONSE RATE TO A QUESTIONNAIRE

One means of reducing the bias in the response to a questionnaire is to identify the individual questionnaires by name or number and keep track of the questionnaires that are returned. Then follow-ups can be mailed to improve the response rate. Unfortunately, many questionnaires have to be confidential and, in those situations, this plan cannot be used.

There are two other means of maximizing the response rate to a questionnaire: 1) using a cover letter to convince the potential respondents to return the completed questionnaire and 2) using a questionnaire that is efficient and requires a minimum of reading and writing by the respondent. In Chapter 6, suggestions were given to provide an efficient questionnaire that would minimize the effort required by the respondent.

A cover letter is extremely important. Each recipient cannot be met personally, so the cover letter is your introduction to the people and the only means you have to convince them to complete and return the questionnaire. Therefore, you must provide the reader with the benefits that he or she will obtain by participating in the study. Even if the benefits are very indirect, the reader must be convinced that it is worth his or her time to fill out the questionnaire. It is also helpful to have the cover letter cosigned by someone known and respected by the people receiving the questionnaire. For example, if you are surveying doctors in a state, the head of the state medical association or a very prominent doctor in the state could add credibility to the value of your study by cosigning the cover letter.

Another suggestion to help improve the response rate is to send a follow-up postcard to all people who were sent a questionnaire. If they have already sent their questionnaires back, you thank them for their participation. If they have not, your note will serve as a reminder. This may help forgetful or busy people who have laid the questionnaire aside and need to have their memories jogged.

One final point: how will the respondent return the questionnaire to you? Providing a stamped, self-addressed return envelope will increase the rate of return, because it will minimize the effort of the respondent.

The main reason for working so carefully to maximize the questionnaire response rate is to minimize the bias that may be present when there is not a total response to the questionnaire. The greater the response rate, the less chance that bias will be present to influence your conclusions. Several authors (references 2, 3, 4, 5, and 9) also discuss the problems inherent in volunteer and questionnaire samples.

Figure 8.1 shows the cover letter sent along with the questionnaire presented in Project 6.2. Official College of Pharmacy stationary was used and the letter was signed by all researchers involved in the study. The letter clearly explains the purpose of this study and informs readers that only 15 minutes of their time is required. The fact that the results will be published is an indirect

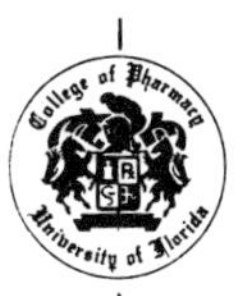

UNIVERSITY OF FLORIDA • J. HILLIS MILLER HEALTH CENTER • GAINESVILLE
COLLEGE OF PHARMACY (Box J-4) 32610

Dear Pharmacist:

Many hospitals maintain a formulary of drugs available for use within their institutions. Policies and procedures for operation of these formularies vary considerably from institution to institution, some being more or less restrictive than others. The College of Pharmacy at the University of Florida is conducting a nationwide survey of all pharmacies in short-term hospitals in an attempt to learn more about certain of these policies and procedures.

Specifically, we are interested in those areas related to selection and interchange of drug products which are chemically equivalent (generically equivalent) and also those which are <u>not</u> chemically but are therapeutically equivalent. The enclosed questionnaire has been designed to allow us to categorize the individual policy approaches to these areas and also to explore attitudes about such policies. Even if you are not currently involved in therapeutic substitution, your responses are necessary to complete our data base.

You can greatly assist us in this research by taking approximately 15 minutes to fill out the questionnaire and returning it in the postage paid envelope which is enclosed no later than November 21. The survey is completely anonymous and there is no way your name or the name of your hospital can be ascertained from the completed questionnaire. We anticipate publication of the data so it can be used by all hospital pharmacists. It is important that your answers are accurate since one of our ultimate goals is to stimulate the drafting and adoption of guidelines concerning these aspects of formulary operation.

Thank you in advance for helping with this research.

Sincerely,

Paul L. Doering, M.S.
Assistant Professor

Deborah L. Klapp, R.Ph.
Adjunct Clinical Instructor

William C. McCormick, Ph.D.
Associate Professor

Wayne L. Russell, Pharm.D.
Clinical Practitioner

EQUAL EMPLOYMENT OPPORTUNITY/AFFIRMATIVE ACTION EMPLOYER

Figure 8.1 Cover letter for questionnaire.

Dear Director of Pharmacy:

Recently we mailed you a questionnaire asking for your participation in an important survey about therapeutic substitution.

If you already returned the questionnaire, please consider this card a "thank you" for your valuable help.

If you have not had a chance to return the completed form yet, could you do so as soon as possible?

Sincerely,

Paul L. Doering

Paul L. Doering
Assistant Professor

Figure 8.2 Follow-up postcard.

benefit of participation, in that respondents can see how they compare with their peers.

Figure 8.2 shows the reminder postcard sent to the pharmacists about 10 days after the questionnaire was mailed. Both the letter and follow-up card are printed in the same colors as those of the questionnaire.

Finally, a prestamped return envelope was provided in which the respondents could return their completed questionnaires.

This questionnaire was very well done. Even so, only 39% of the 6326 pharmacists who received the questionnaire responded. For this particular study, the response rate was deemed acceptable and, in fact, was slightly higher than expected. A low response rate had been expected because many pharmacists would not be interested in the topic and, hence, would not be motivated to respond. Also, the sensitivity of some questions regarding the legality of certain practices would make some people uneasy, in which case they might decide not to participate.

8.10 EVALUATING BIAS

One technique for evaluating the bias in a questionnaire sample requires keeping track of which questionnaires are returned. Then, a random sample of the non-respondents is chosen and these people are contacted a second time. This second contact is carried out in such a way (phone call or personal visit) as to guarantee a response to the questionnaire. A comparison of the responses on the initial return to the second set of responses should show whether any biases were present in the initial responses. If the results of both samples are similar, the researcher may conclude that no biases were present. If the results differ, the researcher may be able to determine which biases are present and in which direction they occur.

Another method of evaluating bias can be used if demographic information is available on all people who receive the questionnaire. Suppose that all doctors in a state medical association are being sent questionnaires. The state association may know the breakdown of doctors by age, sex, location, and type of practice. This information also can be obtained from the questionnaires of respondents, and the overall percentages of respondents can be compared to the entire universe for differences. This technique is valid only for identified demographic factors. Other important personality or attitudinal biases cannot be evaluated by this method.

8.11 WHAT SAMPLING SCHEME FOR YOUR PROJECT?

For the research project whose objective you listed in Chapter 2, evaluate the various sampling schemes available and answer the following questions:

- Which of the four types of sampling schemes (simple random sampling, stratified, cluster, systematic) will be most appropriate for my research project? Should a combination of methods be used?
- Is it possible to employ the appropriate sampling scheme for my research project?
- Will the sample of experimental units I select using the chosen sampling scheme be representative of the entire universe? What biases may be present?
- If biases are present, how may they influence the conclusions that I may draw?

8.12 KEY POINTS

This chapter discussed the importance of striving for a representative sample from the universe so that the conclusions drawn can be extrapolated to the entire universe. The researcher should try to use one of the four types of probability samples—random, stratified, cluster, and systematic. However, in most research projects, a true representative sample cannot be taken. In these instances, potential biases should be identified and controlled for, if possible.

8.13 THE NEXT STEP

The next step in your research design is to determine the sample size you will need to achieve the research objective. In some studies, this procedure is relatively straightforward and yields an accurate estimate. In other, more complex designs, this task becomes quite difficult. However, you should obtain some information about needed sample size before beginning the study. It can be frustrating at the completion of a study to find out that the chosen sample size was too small to achieve the research objective or that much more time was spent collecting data than actually was needed. These frustrations can be avoided by the proper evaluation of sample size needs before the data collection begins.

REFERENCES

1. Berkson, J. 1946. Limitations of the application of fourfold table analysis to hospital data. *Biometric Bulletin* 2: 47–53.
2. Roberts, R. S., Spitzer, W. O., Delmore, T., and Sackett, D. L. 1978. An empirical demonstration of Berkson's bias. *Journal of Chronic Diseases* 31: 119–128.
3. Colton, T. 1974. *Statistics in medicine*. Boston: Little, Brown.
4. Rimm, A. A., Hartz, A. J., Kalbfleisch, J. H., Anderson, A. J., and Hoffmann, R. G. 1980. *Basic biostatistics in medicine and epidemiology*. New York: Appleton-Century-Crofts.
5. Feinstein, A. R. 1977. *Clinical biostatistics*. St. Louis: Mosby. Ch. 6, 7, 11, 12.
6. Feinstein, A. R. 1971. Clinical biostatistics X: Sources of "transition bias" in cohort statistics. *Clin. Pharmacol. Ther*. 12: 704–721.
7. Feinstein, A. R. 1971. Clinical biostatistics XI: Sources of "chronology bias" in cohort statistics. *Clin. Pharmacol. Ther*. 12: 864–879.
8. Feinstein, A. R. 1973. Clinical biostatistics XXII: The role of randomization in sampling, testing, allocation, and credulous idolatry (Part 1). *Clin. Pharmacol. Ther*. 14: 601–615.
9. Feinstein, A. R. 1971. Clinical biostatistics VII: The rancid sample, the tilted target, and the medical poll-bearer. *Clin. Pharmacol. Ther*. 12: 134–150.
10. Levy, P. S., and Lemeshaw, S. 1980. *Sampling for health professionals*. Belmont, Calif.: Lifetime Learning.
11. Mendenhall, W., Ott, L., and Scheaffer, R. L. 1971. *Elementary survey sampling*. Belmont, Calif.: Duxbury.
12. Cochran, W. G. 1963. *Sampling techniques*. New York: Wiley.
13. Raj, D. 1968. *Sampling theory*. New York: McGraw-Hill.

CHAPTER **9**

The Matter of Sample Size Determination

9.1 INTRODUCTION

When you are in the market for a new car, you go to many showrooms and listen to a salesman in each extoll the virtues of his brand. You then evaluate their claims and try to determine which car will best meet your needs, provide reliable performance, and still be in reasonably good shape in five years. If there is a car that you really like but that you believe will fall apart when it is five years old, you will probably look elsewhere.

In the world of biomedical research, consider yourself a salesperson trying to sell a product to a granting agency, which is the consumer. The granting agency (consumer) has to evaluate many grant proposals submitted by different researchers (salespeople) and determine which projects it should fund (buy).

The granting agency will evaluate each proposal in two very general areas. First, it will look at the scientific merit of the proposed research and the quality of the research team in conducting the research. Second, it will evaluate the ability of the project to reach its desired objective in five years (or whatever the length of time for which the proposal is funded). You may have a great research project outlined for which you are requesting \$1 million in funding for five years. However, if the granting agency feels that the research requires 200 subjects to achieve the research objective and that you can study only 50 subjects in that time, funding probably will not be granted. Although you have a good idea that should be investigated, the granting agency would be spending \$1 million in five years and would not have the desired question answered. Would you buy a new car that gets the best gas mileage and has the most interior room and best looks if you felt that it would be ready for the junk pile in five years, while its less desirable competition would still be in good condition and have many more highway miles left?

Increased granting competition will require even better sales jobs by researchers who hope to get their research projects funded. One of the most important and direct questions that a granting agency will ask of any researcher submitting a grant proposal is to justify the choice of the sample size made in the proposal.

If you state in the grant proposal that 50 people will be studied because that is the practical maximum number of participants that you think will be available, the proposal probably will be rejected unless you can convince the review panel that this number of participants is large enough to achieve the research objective scientifically.

9.2 KNOW YOUR PRACTICAL SAMPLE SIZE

You have a good idea before beginning the research project of what the *practical* limitations are on your sample size. In Project 3.1, in which the researcher studied patients undergoing gastric partition surgery, he or she might schedule one surgery each week. After accounting for vacations, holidays, sick time, out-of-town travels, and patients who are uncooperative, the researcher may expect to obtain data on 30 patients per year. You must be very careful not to be too optimistic in the number of subjects that you realistically can be expected to obtain. If this study is to run three years and you convince the granting agency to fund your research because 90 people studied over three years are enough to achieve the research objective, and if you study only 60 people because you overestimated the available pool of participants, you will be in trouble with the granting agency for failure to comply with the proposal you submitted and had funded. If you get nervous because you will not make your stated sample size and hence include people who are either too old, have other illnesses, or should otherwise be excluded, you run the risk of introducing biases into the data, which could lead to erroneous conclusions being drawn. Thus, you *must* be very confident of obtaining the sample size promised in the proposal.

9.3 HOW TO SELL YOUR SAMPLE SIZE

After you have determined the practical sample size that you are confident you can obtain, you must sell this sample size to the granting agency. To do so, you must convince the granting agency that this sample size is adequate (large enough) to achieve the research objective. You will need to restate the research objective as a research hypothesis, usually in terms of appropriate population parameters. Then you must answer a number of mathematical questions about the data to be collected and the research hypothesis to be answered. These questions will be discussed in this chapter, and examples showing how to answer them will be given in the next chapter. The answers to these questions, along with information about the research design and type of response variable included in the analysis, can be put into an appropriate mathematical formula that will yield the estimated sample size *needed* to prove the research hypothesis and, hence, achieve the research objective. The sample size needed to prove the research hypothesis statistically should agree closely with the practical sample available. If the needed sample size is less than what is available (which is seldom the case), you and the granting agency should be pleased.

However, if the needed sample size is larger than what is available, you must make some hard decisions. Can you adjust the goals of the study to be less specific, so that a smaller sample size will suffice? Can some aspect of the research design be improved, such as by the use of repeated measures, to increase the amount of information obtained from the P-sample? Should you drop this project completely and find another project with more chance of success? Or should you submit the proposal as it is and take a chance that the agency will fund the project as it stands? This decision is never an easy one to make and must be made on an individual project basis.

You must obtain this information *before* submitting the proposal so that you can evaluate the chances of 1) obtaining funding and 2) achieving the research objective by proving the research hypothesis.

9.4 SAMPLE SIZE ESTIMATION IN THESES AND DISSERTATIONS

If, instead of submitting a grant proposal, you are a graduate student carrying out a research project as part of a thesis or dissertation, it is equally important to consider the needed sample size before beginning data collection. However, it is not as critical to achieve the needed sample size in practice for a thesis or dissertation, especially at the Master's level, as it is for an expensive, multi-year grant. The objective of many graduate programs requiring research projects is to have the student learn the research process rather than to have him or her prove some hypothesis statistically. If the needed sample size greatly exceeds the available sample, the student and his or her committee can determine whether the project still should be carried out, even if statistical significance is not obtained. The student still will be learning about research design, getting approval from the committee for the protection of human subjects (if necessary), experiencing the problems inherent in actually collecting the data, and carrying out the analysis of research data. The only change in plans would be to consider the project as a pilot study with no hard conclusions required or expected.

I have seen cases in which a graduate committee enthusiastically endorses a student's proposal because the idea is good and because new information can be obtained on some topic. The student, thinking he or she is on the right track to get excellent results that will please the committee, goes about collecting the available data and then analyzes them. When the results are not statistically significant, the committee criticizes the student, blaming him or her for doing poor research. The student now is confused, not knowing how things went wrong, and loses interest in research.

Instead, the student and the committee should have estimated the approximate sample size needed to prove the research hypothesis. If the needed sample size was not available, the committee would have been warned that statistically significant results were unlikely. Then, the student and the committee together could have made an informed decision to redesign the study or to proceed with the planned project, treating it as a pilot study.

This area of sample size estimation is probably the most important in improving the attitude of novice researchers toward conducting more research. They must be helped to evaluate what constitutes a valid research project *before* it is completed. The committee should help the student anticipate possible conclusions, consider the chances of each occurring, and decide whether these conclusions will be acceptable. If biomedical researchers hope to increase the quantity of research and improve its quality, they must encourage students to become interested and actively engage in research. To accomplish this end, committees must *teach* students the fundamentals of conducting good research instead of expecting them to *learn* research methods simply by doing and then being quizzed on what they have done.

9.5 THE VALUE OF THE COMPUTED SAMPLE SIZE

A single number can be computed that represents the sample size necessary to achieve the desired results of the research hypothesis. What is the value of this single number?

First, you will see in the later examples that by changing your answers to some questions asked of you, you can change the needed sample size quite a bit. This fact should make you wonder whether you might be able somehow to show statistically that a sample size of 10 is needed if that is your available sample. The answer is that you can do so. However, although you can arrive statistically at a sample size similar to your available small sample size, you must be able to defend the answers that you gave to the questions asked, and this part may prove difficult.

On the other hand, no one single sample size estimate is the exact sample size needed to achieve your research objective. The questions you must consider can be answered only approximately, and hence, the resulting sample size is approximate. It is meant to give you a ballpark figure. Will about 20, 200, or 2000 experimental units be sufficient to achieve the research objective?

There is nothing wrong with making a few sample size estimations by changing the answers to some questions. This approach will provide you with a range of needed sample sizes. Remember that whichever sample size or range of sample sizes you choose, you must justify that choice with your answers to the questions involved.

Keeping these constraints in mind, let us now take a look at the questions you must consider and answer to arrive at a needed sample size estimate.

9.6 STATEMENT OF THE RESEARCH OBJECTIVE

The first step in determining the sample size is to restate the research objective, usually, but not necessarily, in terms of the appropriate population parameters. Remember that the parameter P denotes the percentage of observations that fall into a particular category of a nominal response variable, ξ denotes the median of an ordinal response variable, μ denotes the mean of a numerical response variable, and σ^2 denotes the variability of a numerical response variable.

Project 3.2 had as its objective **to estimate the percentage of generically substituted prescriptions from all pharmacies in the state of Florida for a previous chosen month.** The research objective in this study is to estimate accurately P, defined as the true, and unknown, generic substitution rate for the state of Florida for that month. If, instead, the objective had been **to compare independent and chain pharmacies to see if their generic substitution rates differed,** the research objective would be to compare statistically P_I and P_C, which denote the true substitution rates for independent and chain pharmacies, respectively.

Project 3.3 had as its objective **to determine whether the breathing of people either with or without breathing problems changes when they are exposed to SO_2.** Several factors were to be studied in this project and several response variables were to be measured, so there may be a number of research objectives to evaluate. For example, define μ_N as the true average FEV_1 of all normals after breathing SO_2. Similarly, μ_A represents the analogous parameter for asthmatics. Then, one research objective would be to determine whether the average FEV_1 differs between normals and asthmatics after they have breathed air and SO_2 for three hours; or, does $\mu_N = \mu_A$? Another research objective might be to estimate the true average rate of change in FEV_1 in normals during a three-hour period. The parameter μ could designate the true average rate of change, and we would be interested in accurately estimating μ.

In both Project 3.2 and Project 3.3, two research objectives were given. For each project, one research objective was written to estimate a parameter and the other objective was to determine whether two parameters have identical values. This second research objective would be answered by the use of some statistical *test* of an appropriately stated hypothesis in terms of the population parameters.

In general, a research objective always is of one of two types: 1) to *estimate* accurately a parameter (such as P) or some combination of parameters (such as $P_1 - P_2$), or 2) to *test* a hypothesis about a parameter or a set of parameters. The sample size will be influenced by the type of research objective and the type of parameter (or parameters) in which you are interested.

We shall discuss the considerations necessary in the determination of sample size for both estimation and hypothesis testing situations. However, for both types, you must provide a measure of variability, σ^2, for a numerical response variable. So, before looking at estimation and hypothesis testing considerations, we shall look at how variability influences the research objective and see how to estimate the variability for a numerical response variable.

9.7 MEASURING VARIABILITY

If the response variable is numerical and we wish to make an inference about the parameter μ or $\mu_1 - \mu_2$, we must be able to provide an estimate of the variability of the response variable. This estimate of σ is necessary whether our objective involves parameter estimation or hypothesis testing.

As an example, suppose a researcher wishes to study the relationship between type of drug (Drug A versus Drug B) and heart rate. Five people are assigned to receive Drug A and five other people to receive Drug B. If the resulting heart rates are as shown in Table 9.1, one could easily conclude that people on Drug A had a lower average heart rate than did those on Drug B.

In the real world, however, response variable measurements are never that consistent. Another possible set of heart rates is presented in Table 9.2.

In both examples, the average heart rate of people on Drug A is 45 and the average heart rate of Drug B is 50. However, in Table 9.2 it is much more difficult to tell whether there is a true difference in heart rates treated by Drugs A and B

Table 9.1 Heart rates of people on drugs A and B

Drug A	*Drug B*
45	50
45	50
45	50
45	50
45	50

Table 9.2 Heart rates of people on drugs A and B

Drug A	*Drug B*
42	59
48	48
40	50
50	41
45	52

than in Table 9.1. The variability of the numbers in Table 9.2 clouds the issue of whether a drug difference truly exists.

In general, the more variability present in the response variable, the more difficult it becomes to answer a particular research question, such as whether two drugs are equivalent. Thus, as the variability increases, the sample size must be increased to enable you to draw an inference about an entire population of response variable measurements. Trying to determine the variability in response variable measurements can present a problem: often we do not know beforehand how variable the measurements will be. At least, we should have an idea of the approximate range of the response variable. The **range** is defined as the difference between the largest and smallest possible measurements in the population. Then the **standard deviation,** σ, for a population can be estimated as one-fourth of the range; that is, $\sigma \approx$ range/4. This approximation is very accurate and only requires the researcher to estimate the range. In the examples in the next chapter, we shall see how to do so.

9.8 PARAMETER ESTIMATION

The objective of a research project may be to estimate some parameter, as "to estimate the generic substitution rate, P, for prescriptions in the state of Florida," or "to estimate the average difference, $\mu_1 - \mu_2$, in heart rate between people on two different doses of a drug," or "to estimate average potency, μ, retained by a drug as a function of the type of storage container, storage temperature, length of storage, and amount of drug stored." In each of these examples, we wish to measure accurately some population parameter when no factors are present, as in the first example, or in the presence of some factors, as in the other examples. In each example, the population parameter is unknown, because the entire population cannot be sampled. Thus, the objective is to estimate that parameter as accurately as possible with the available sample data.

In any estimation problem, the researcher needs to arrive at both a **point estimate** and an **interval estimate.** The point estimate is the best guess of the true value of the parameter you wish to estimate, while the interval estimate gives a measure of the accuracy of that point estimate by providing an interval that should contain the true value of the parameter of interest. **Bound on error** is another measure of the accuracy of a parameter estimate. It is the same as the interval estimate.

For example, we may have collected data to estimate the true generic substitution rate in the state of Florida. The computed point estimate may be 6% and the bound on error 2%. Thus the best guess of the true generic substitution rate (P), based on the observed data, is 6%, and although the estimate probably is not totally correct, we are confident that it is within 2% of the correct rate: that is, the interval estimate for P is 4% to 8%. Thus, in any research project involving parameter estimation, we must strive for a reasonable interval estimate (or bound on error). In this example, a bound on error of 30% is unreasonably large, while a bound of .1% is probably unnecessarily small. The sample size will influence the size of the interval estimate: the larger your sample size, the smaller the interval estimate. Thus, the sample size should be chosen that will yield a reasonable bound for your interval estimate.

The point and interval estimates are combined to form what is called a confidence interval. A 95% confidence interval is most commonly computed, but 90%, 99%, or any other confidence interval can be computed also. The choice of confidence coefficient, like the sample size, influences the size of the interval estimate. The term 90%, 95%, or 99% is called the **confidence coefficient** and reflects our confidence that the computed interval will contain the parameter of interest. A 95% confidence interval for the generic substitution example means that if samples of a constant size were taken repeatedly and if for each sample a 95% confidence interval were computed, 95% of the computed intervals would contain the true value of the parameter P. Thus, if 100 researchers each randomly sampled 50 different adults, measured their heart rates, and computed 95% confidence intervals for the true average adult heart rate, *about* 95 of them would have intervals containing the true, unknown, average value. The others did not make any errors in their research methodology: the fact that the true value of the parameter lies outside their computed intervals merely happened by chance. Obviously, a 99% confidence interval is wider than a 95% confidence interval, which is, in turn, wider than a 90% confidence interval. You should choose the confidence coefficient that will be most acceptable for your particular goal.

Thus, if we choose 1) the confidence coefficient and 2) the desired size of the interval estimate, we can compute the sample size needed to achieve those results. Actual computations for some simple designs are given in the next chapter. For other designs, a professional statistician should be consulted.

For a numerical response variable, the variability must be determined, as we discussed earlier, and the size of the confidence interval is influenced by the size of σ.

Computational formulas for the parameters P, $P_1 - P_2$, μ, and $\mu_1 - \mu_2$ can be found in references 1 through 3, as well as in most other introductory statistics textbooks. Examples of computing the sample size for an estimation problem are given in the next chapter.

9.9 TESTING A HYPOTHESIS ABOUT A SET OF PARAMETERS

The objective of a research project may be to answer some question such as: "Is the generic substitution rate for prescriptions the same in Florida as it is in the rest of the nation?" or "Is there an effect on either asthmatics or non-asthmatics of increasing sulfur in the air?" or "Is the rate of epileptic seizures less in people who use Drug X than in those who use Drug Y?" Rather than trying to estimate parameters, we are looking for a *yes* or *no* answer to each of these questions. Again, the appropriate population parameters would be defined and the research objective to be tested usually would be stated in terms of a hypothesis about these parameters. Then the appropriate statistical test would be computed from the collected data and a conclusion could be drawn about the stated question.

9.9.1 Testing Steps

In any hypothesis-testing situation, there are several steps to perform. They are as follows:

1. Determine the null hypothesis (H_0).
2. Determine the alternative hypothesis (H_a).
3. Determine a suitable significance level and power for the statistical test.
4. Choose and compute the test statistic.
5. Make a conclusion.

We shall now introduce steps 1, 2, and 3. (For a detailed discussion of steps 4 and 5, see reference 7.)

9.9.2 Null and Alternative Hypotheses

The null and alternative hypotheses are stated in such a way that you can show your research objective. You will see as we go through the later chapters that the null (H_0) and alternative (H_a) hypotheses are usually, though not necessarily, stated in terms of appropriate population parameters. We might test a hypothesis to determine whether a single parameter could equal some constant. An example would be to determine whether the generic substitution rate in the state of Florida is substantially different from 10%: that is, is $P = .10$ or $P \neq .10$? Or, we may wish to compare a set of parameters to determine whether their values are very similar. An example would be to determine whether the generic substitution rate for independent pharmacies (denoted P_I) is equal to the rate for chain pharmacies (P_C): that is, does $P_I = P_C$ or $P_I \neq P_C$?

All hypotheses that we consider for H_0 are stated as some equality, whereas H_a usually is stated as an inequality. For example, suppose two drugs, A and B, are being compared to determine which one can cure more people with a certain illness. We are interested in comparing P_A and P_B, the true, and unknown, cure rates for Drugs A and B, respectively. Before the study is conducted, no information is available as to which drug, if either, is superior. Thus, H_0 would be expressed as $H_0: P_A = P_B$ to indicate that we are assuming that the drugs are comparable in curing this illness. H_a can be stated in a number of ways, depending on what we are trying to prove. If we have no preconceived idea as to which drug may be superior and we wish to detect any difference between the two drugs, H_a would be $H_a: P_A \neq P_B$. H_a is called a **two-tail alternative** in this case, and we would be able to conclude that either Drug A or Drug B was superior, if the data support either conclusion.

On the other hand, suppose we have developed Drug B and it is considered a successful development only if it is superior to existing Drug A. Or suppose a hospital currently uses Drug A and is considering switching to Drug B only if it is superior to Drug A. In that case, $H_a: P_B > P_A$, meaning that we are interested only in showing that the cure rate for Drug B is higher than that for Drug A. This case is called a **one-tail alternative** and can be used only if the researcher is interested intuitively in showing a difference in one direction. It is important to note that H_0 and H_a are established *before* we observe the data: that is, the data generally should not be used to determine the research hypotheses. Statistical tests are available to test hypotheses determined by observation of the data, but we shall not discuss these techniques. A similar argument would be used for establishing H_0 and H_a for any set of parameters, as we shall see throughout the rest of the book.

9.9.3 Significance Level and Power

After the data are collected, we compute an appropriate test statistic and then determine whether to accept H_0 as being true or reject it as being false. Regardless of which decision we make, we must be concerned with whether or not the correct decision was made. The four possible outcomes for a statistical test of a hypothesis are shown in Figure 9.1.

If H_0 is accepted as being true based on the observed measurements and it really is true, then a correct decision was made. Likewise, if H_0 is rejected for H_a and this situation is the true one, then a correct decision again was made. However, if H_0 is rejected and it is really true, then what is called a *Type I error* was committed. If H_0 is accepted as being true when H_a is true, then a *Type II error* has been committed. Thus, whenever your decision is to reject H_0, you must be aware that a Type I error may have been made, whereas if your conclusion is to accept H_0, you must be concerned with committing a Type II error. Your concern about making each of these errors can be measured by a computation of their probability of occurrence. When the decision is to reject H_0 in favor of H_a, the probability of committing a Type I error is defined as the **significance level of the statistical test** and is denoted as p or α. (Note that although p and α both represent significance level, there is a difference in their meaning. See reference 7.) We can measure the significance level of a test easily and know how confident we are in the decision to reject H_0. Note that the parameter P is denoted by a capital letter, while the significance level p is denoted by a lower-case letter to distinguish these two terms clearly.

		Decision based on data	
		Accept H_0	Reject H_0
Real life Situation	H_0 true	Correct decision	Type I error
	H_a true	Type II error	Correct decision

Figure 9.1 Four outcomes for a statistical test.

A Type II error can be committed only when our decision is to accept H_0 as being true when H_a really is true. As you will see, H_0 always is stated as an equality in terms of the appropriate population parameters, whereas H_a generally is stated as an inequality. The probability of a Type II error, denoted β, can be computed only for an exact alternative hypothesis and would differ for each possible alternative. Thus, we must decide on an appropriate alternative that we want to detect if it really exists. Then, for that particular H_a, β can be computed. The **power** of a statistical test is defined as its ability to lead to the rejection of H_0, if H_0 is really false. The power of a test would equal $1 - \beta$ for a particular alternative.

For example, in the comparison of the generic substitution rates of independent and chain pharmacies, the hypothesis to test is $H_0: P_I = P_C$ (or $P_I - P_C = 0$) versus $H_a: P_I \neq P_C$ (or $P_I - P_C \neq 0$). We now must consider how great a difference between P_I and P_C we should show. With a large enough sample size, a difference of 1% can be shown to be statistically significant. However, if this difference is too small to be meaningful, that large a sample size is unnecessary. Is a 2% difference important, or 5%, or 10%? In any hypothesis-testing problem, the researcher must decide how great a difference between the parameters is important. Then, for that exact alternative, β can be determined. The smaller the difference that is important, the larger is the sample size needed to show it.

Before we begin our study, we would like to feel confident that both α and β will be sufficiently small, because they represent the probability of making an erroneous conclusion. As the sample size is increased, more information is obtained, and each of these probabilities is reduced. Thus, once we choose a suitable α and β (for a particular alternative), we can compute the sample size needed to test the stated hypothesis. For a fixed sample size, increasing α will result in a reduction of β, and vice versa. Some researchers prefer to use a very small α level for a statistical test and do not realize that the result is to increase β. Examples of determining the sample size for testing hypotheses about certain parameters are given in the next chapter.

As with estimation, the variability of numerical response variable measurements influences the sample size needed to test a hypothesis, and the range also is used to estimate standard deviation, as we showed earlier. Again, the more variability present in the response variable, the larger is the sample size required to reject H_0 in favor of H_a. Additional information on estimating the sample size required for testing the hypotheses $H_0: P_1 = P_2$ on $H_0: \mu_1 - \mu_2$ can be found elsewhere (references 4,5).

9.10 CLINICAL VERSUS STATISTICAL SIGNIFICANCE

You may wonder why it is so important to compute the needed sample size before beginning the data collection. The reason is that you want the results of the study that are shown statistically also to be clinically important to you.

	Antihypertensive drug A	Antihypertensive drug B
Average systolic blood pressure $n_1 = n_2 = 500$	140.2 mm Hg	140.3 mm Hg

$p < .001$

Highly significant!

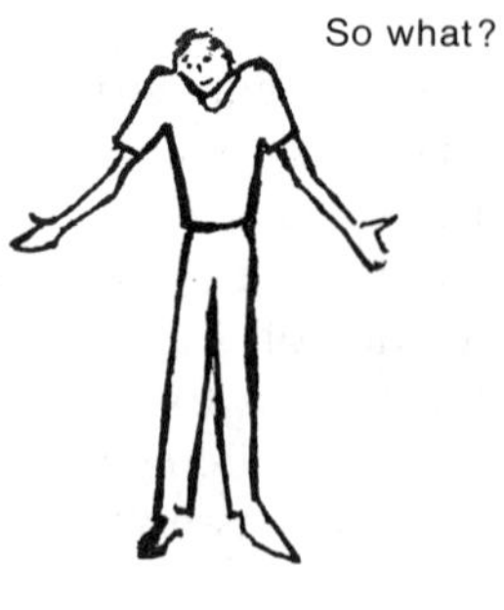

	Antihypertensive drug A	Antihypertensive drug B
Average systolic blood pressure $n_1 = n_2 = 10$	124.6 mm Hg	149.8 mm Hg

$p < .31$

Not statistically significant!

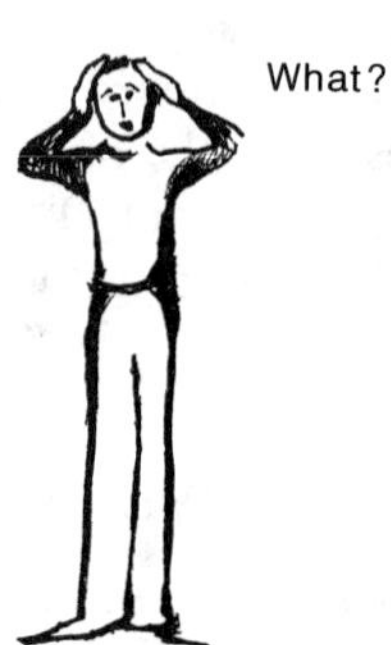

Figure 9.2 Statistically and clinically important differences.

The results of some studies whose test of hypothesis is statistically significant sometimes produce the reaction "so what?" if the proven difference between the factor levels is small. In other studies in which the results of a statistical test are not significant, the researcher sometimes feels that an important clinical difference nonetheless has been shown. Both situations are the result of improper consideration of sample size needs for the study. You must realize that no two factor levels are truly equivalent. Even if the true average systolic blood pressure for all people on one antihypertensive drug is 140.2 mm Hg and the true mean for a second drug is 140.3 mm Hg, a statistically significant difference could be shown if the sample sizes were large enough. However, this small difference may not be clinically important. A clinically important difference should be established first by an appropriate alternative hypothesis and then the sample size computed to show significance for that difference. Instead, some researchers might collect a larger P-sample than needed to show a difference that was not important.

Alternatively, the researcher may feel that the observed difference is clinically important, even though it was not determined to be statistically significant. This result would occur if the sample size were too small to show the desired difference. This problem could have been determined before any data were collected. Thus, the sample size determinations are important to assure the researcher that the results will be significant *both* statistically *and* clinically.

Most granting agencies require a researcher submitting a grant proposal to justify the choice of sample size. The agency wants to be sure, before providing substantial funding for a research project, that the sample size is large enough to prove the research hypothesis with much confidence. Also, it wants assurance that the researcher is not collecting a great deal more data than are necessary and, hence, is not asking for more money than is needed to achieve the research objective. Thus, it is important to justify the choice of sample size statistically rather than by stating, "This is all that I can afford," or "This is all that is available."

9.11 ESTIMATION VERSUS HYPOTHESIS TESTING

For each research objective to evaluate, you must decide whether you are interested in estimating a parameter (or set of parameters) or in testing some stated hypothesis about the parameters. In most cases, a hypothesis-testing procedure is chosen, probably because hypothesis testing is stressed more in statistics courses and because it is much more prevalent in the scientific literature. Some statisticians present an interesting argument against the use of hypothesis-testing procedures, claiming that no two treatments (or any set of factor levels) are exactly equal. They point out that, given a large enough sample, any null hypothesis eventually can be rejected. What is of interest is the *magnitude* of the difference, and this question is not answered by the test of a hypothesis. For more information on this point of view, see reference 6.

Let us now take a more detailed look at estimating the sample size for the estimation and testing of various population parameters. In the next chapter, we shall look at estimating and testing hypotheses about the parameters P, $P_1 - P_2$, μ, and $\mu_1 - \mu_2$.

9.12 KEY POINTS

This chapter has introduced one of the most important concepts of research design—determining the sample size needed to achieve the research objective. You must answer several important questions before you can determine the needed sample size. Some of these questions may prove difficult, and you can make only an educated guess as to the answers. Thus, the computed sample size is an approximation that will give you an idea of how many observations are needed to achieve the research objective.

After you have determined the needed sample size, you can compare this number to the practical sample size available and decide whether to proceed with the study as planned, make some changes in the research design, or drop the project and start over.

In the next chapter, examples will show how to determine the sample size. They will familiarize you with the questions that must be answered and show how to make appropriate decisions once the sample size has been determined.

REFERENCES

1. McClave, J. T., and Dietrich, F. H. II. 1979. *Statistics*. San Francisco: Dellen.

2. Mendenhall, W. 1979. *Introduction to probability and statistics*. Belmont, Calif.: Duxbury.

3. Dixon, W. J., and Massey, F. J., Jr. 1969. *Introduction to statistical analysis*. New York: McGraw-Hill.

4. Walpole, R. E., and Myers, R. H. 1972. *Probability and statistics for engineers and scientists*. New York: Macmillan.

5. Fleiss, J. L. 1981. *Statistical methods for rates and proportions*. New York: Wiley.

6. Chew, V. 1980. Testing differences among means: Correct interpretation and some alternatives. *Hort. Science* 15: 4, 467–470.

7. Marks, R. 1982. *Analyzing Research Data*. Belmont, Calif.: Lifetime Learning Publications.

CHAPTER 10

Determining the Proper Sample Size

10.1 INTRODUCTION

In the last chapter, we introduced the considerations necessary to determine the needed sample size for a research project. Sample size determination sometimes is very complex and, even for relatively simple research designs, can be difficult. The reason is that you must answer several questions to determine the sample size, and arriving at accurate answers may be difficult.

Also, the computed sample size is not a magical number guaranteed to answer all your questions. It is an approximate figure for the number of needed experimental units. By changing the answers to your questions, you can determine different sample sizes. Thus, the accuracy of the determined sample size is related to the accuracy of the answers that you can provide to the questions.

You also should remember that using the determined sample size *does not* guarantee that the research objective will be achieved, but indicates that your chances of achieving it are satisfactorily high. Likewise, using a smaller than desirable sample size does not guarantee that the research objective cannot be obtained, but indicates that the chances of doing so may be low.

10.2 QUESTIONS TO ANSWER IN DETERMINING SAMPLE SIZE

In any research project, the answers to several questions are essential to determining sample size.

First, if the response variable is numerical, either discrete or continuous, the amount of variability in the response variable measurements must be measured. The more variable are the measurements, the more difficult it is to achieve the research objective, and hence, the larger is the sample size that is required.

Second, the type of inference to be made and the magnitude of the inference must be determined. In the last chapter, we showed that the two general types of inference that can be drawn are estimation and hypothesis testing. If you wish to estimate a parameter, you must determine a suitable bound on error. The more accuracy desired in the estimated parameter (determined by the chosen bound on error), the larger the sample size required. Similarly, for hypothesis testing, the smaller the difference you wish to show between a set of parameters, the larger the required sample size will be.

The third consideration is whether some type of repeated measures or blocking is being employed. As we showed in Chapter 7, a repeated measure or block design can reduce the number of experimental units required for a study. Another consideration is the number of factors and the number of levels of each factor that will be evaluated. After these questions have been answered, an appropriate mathematical formula can be used to determine the sample size. This procedure can be complicated, and a statistician should be consulted, if available. We shall look only at determining the sample size for some simple designs in this chapter.

A practical consideration is the number of experimental units that you can include in the study because of limitations of time, money, and the availability of experimental units. You should compare the computed sample size to the available sample size and then decide whether to proceed with the project or make some changes. You may wish to make changes if the available sample size is much smaller than the sample size needed to achieve the research objective.

Let us now look at some examples of estimating the needed sample size for projects where estimation is the type of inference we wish to make. We then shall use the same examples for hypothesis-testing types of inference to contrast the two types of inference.

10.3 COMPUTING SAMPLE SIZE FOR ESTIMATING THE PARAMETER *P*

Project 10.1 Estimating generic substitution in Florida

Refer to Project 3.2, whose objective was **to estimate the percentage of generically substituted prescriptions, denoted *P*, in the state of Florida for a given month.**

In this example, the response variable is *yes* or *no*, to represent whether a particular prescription (experimental unit) had a generic substitution. Because the response variable is nominal, the usual numerical concept of variability between individual response variable measurements does not apply. However, to select the appropriate sample size, we must decide how accurately we wish to estimate this percentage and with what confidence we wish the confidence interval to contain the true value of the parameter. Obviously, a much larger sample is required to estimate the true percentage to within .5% than would be required at 2%. Suppose we decide to estimate the true percentage to within 2%, with a 95% confidence coefficient. This means that if the resulting sample size is obtained, the bound on error should be about 2%. Furthermore, if samples were taken repeatedly and separate confidence intervals computed for each sample, about 95% of the computed intervals would contain the true value of the parameter P. Alternatively, even though random samples were taken, 5% of the resulting confidence intervals would not contain the true value of the parameter.

For any sample size estimation involving a nominal response variable, we must guess at the value of P. The mathematical equation used to estimate sample size involves the value of P. Obviously, we only can guess the value, because if it were known, the research project would be unnecessary. For this project, we guess that P should be approximately 10%, or $P = .10$. Now that we have the bound chosen at 2% ($B = .02$), the confidence coefficient is 95% ($CC = .95$), and $P = .10$, the needed sample size can be found in Table 10.1. This table results from computing the sample size needed for estimating P using the appropriate mathematical equation for different values of P, CC, and B. Go down the column labeled P until you find a P value of .10. Note that $P = .10$ is listed three times, once each for the confidence coefficients 90%, 95%, and 99%. Because $CC = .95$, use row 29 of the table. Now go across row 29 until you arrive at the column for $B = .02$. The number given, 865, is the sample size needed to meet your requirements in achieving the research objective. Had we chosen $CC = .99$ instead, we would have $n = 1487$; or if we had used a bound of 5%, $B = .05$, we would have $n = 139$. Note that the table only goes up to $P = .5$. The reason is that we can obtain the sample sizes for values greater than .5 from this table by subtracting them from 1. Thus, the same sample sizes would result for an estimation of P if it were about .90 instead of .10.

If you would like to compute a sample size for a value of P, CC, or B not in Table 10.1, the equation to use is

$$n = \frac{Z^2 \times P \times (1 - P)}{B^2} \tag{10.1}$$

where Z is obtained from a table of standard normal values for a particular value of CC. For $CC = .90$, $Z = 1.645$; for $CC = .95$, $Z = 1.96$; and for $CC = .99$, $Z = 2.57$.

Let us look at another example.

Table 10.1 Sample sizes required to estimate P for various confidence coefficients and bounds

			BOUND (B)									
Row	*P*	*CC*	.01	.02	.03	.04	.05	.06	.07	.08	.09	.10
1	0.01	0.90	268	67	30	17	11	8	6	5	4	3
2	0.01	0.95	381	96	43	24	16	11	8	6	5	4
3	0.01	0.99	654	164	73	41	27	19	14	11	9	7
4	0.02	0.90	531	133	59	34	22	15	11	9	7	6
5	0.02	0.95	753	189	84	48	31	21	16	12	10	8
6	0.02	0.99	1295	324	144	81	52	36	27	21	16	13
7	0.03	0.90	788	197	88	50	32	22	17	13	10	8
8	0.03	0.95	1118	280	125	70	45	32	23	18	14	12
9	0.03	0.99	1923	481	214	121	77	54	40	31	24	20
10	0.04	0.90	1040	260	116	65	42	29	22	17	13	11
11	0.04	0.95	1476	369	164	93	60	41	31	24	19	15
12	0.04	0.99	2537	635	282	159	102	71	52	40	32	25
13	0.05	0.90	1286	322	143	81	52	36	27	21	16	13
14	0.05	0.95	1825	457	203	115	73	51	38	29	23	19
15	0.05	0.99	3133	785	349	197	126	88	65	50	39	32
16	0.06	0.90	1527	382	170	96	62	43	32	24	19	16
17	0.06	0.95	2167	542	241	135	87	61	45	34	27	22
18	0.06	0.99	3726	932	414	233	150	104	77	59	46	38
19	0.07	0.90	1762	441	196	111	71	49	36	28	22	18
20	0.07	0.95	2501	626	278	157	101	70	52	40	31	26
21	0.07	0.99	4300	1075	478	269	172	120	88	68	54	43
22	0.08	0.90	1992	498	222	125	80	56	41	32	25	20
23	0.08	0.95	2828	707	315	177	114	79	58	45	35	29
24	0.08	0.99	4862	1216	541	304	195	136	100	76	61	49
25	0.09	0.90	2217	555	247	139	89	62	46	35	28	23
26	0.09	0.95	3147	787	350	197	126	88	65	50	39	32
27	0.09	0.99	5410	1353	602	339	217	151	111	85	67	55
28	0.10	0.90	2436	609	271	153	98	68	50	39	31	25
29	0.10	0.95	3458	865	385	217	139	97	71	55	43	35
30	0.10	0.99	5945	1487	661	372	238	166	122	93	74	60
31	0.11	0.90	2650	663	295	165	106	74	55	42	33	27
32	0.11	0.95	3761	941	418	236	151	105	77	59	47	38
33	0.11	0.99	6467	1617	719	405	259	180	132	102	80	65
34	0.12	0.90	2858	715	318	179	115	80	59	45	36	29
35	0.12	0.95	4057	1015	451	254	163	113	83	64	51	41
36	0.12	0.99	6975	1744	775	436	279	194	143	109	87	70
37	0.13	0.90	3061	766	341	192	123	86	63	48	38	31
38	0.13	0.95	4345	1087	483	272	174	121	89	68	54	44
39	0.13	0.99	7471	1868	831	467	299	208	153	117	93	75
40	0.14	0.90	3259	815	363	204	131	91	67	51	41	33
41	0.14	0.95	4626	1157	514	290	186	129	95	73	58	47
42	0.14	0.99	7953	1989	884	498	319	221	163	125	99	80
43	0.15	0.90	3451	863	384	216	139	96	71	54	43	35
44	0.15	0.95	4899	1225	545	307	196	137	100	77	61	49
45	0.15	0.99	8422	2106	936	527	337	234	172	132	104	85
46	0.20	0.90	4330	1083	482	271	174	121	89	68	54	44
47	0.20	0.95	6147	1537	683	385	246	171	126	97	76	62
48	0.20	0.99	10568	2642	1175	661	423	294	216	166	131	106
49	0.25	0.90	5074	1269	564	313	203	141	104	80	63	51
50	0.25	0.95	7203	1801	801	451	289	201	148	113	89	73
51	0.25	0.99	12385	3097	1377	775	496	345	253	194	153	124
52	0.30	0.90	5683	1421	632	356	228	158	116	89	71	57
53	0.30	0.95	8068	2017	897	505	323	225	165	127	100	81
54	0.30	0.99	13871	3468	1542	867	555	386	284	217	172	139
55	0.35	0.90	6157	1540	685	385	247	172	126	97	77	62
56	0.35	0.95	8740	2185	972	547	350	243	179	137	108	88
57	0.35	0.99	15027	3757	1670	940	602	418	307	235	186	151
58	0.40	0.90	6495	1624	722	406	260	181	133	102	81	65
59	0.40	0.95	9220	2305	1025	577	369	257	189	145	114	93
60	0.40	0.99	15852	3963	1762	991	635	441	324	248	196	159
61	0.45	0.90	6698	1675	745	419	268	187	137	105	83	67
62	0.45	0.95	9508	2377	1057	595	381	265	195	149	118	96
63	0.45	0.99	16348	4087	1817	1022	654	455	334	256	202	164
64	0.50	0.90	6766	1692	752	423	271	188	139	106	84	68
65	0.50	0.95	9605	2402	1068	501	385	267	197	151	119	97
66	0.50	0.99	16513	4129	1835	1033	661	459	337	259	204	166

Project 10.2 Estimation of the percentage of school-age children with breathing problems

A physiologist would like **to estimate the percentage of school-age children in his state with some type of breathing problem,** such as asthma or a particular type of allergy. For this project,

Universe	All school-age children in this state, defined as between the ages of 6 and 18
Experimental unit	Each individual child between the ages of 6 and 18
Response variable	*Yes*, the child has a breathing problem; or *no*, the child has no breathing problem
Population	The collection of *yes* and *no* responses for all children in the universe
U-sample	The collection of children chosen to participate in the study
P-sample	The collection of *yes* and *no* responses for the children included in the study

For this project, as with the generic substitution example discussed previously, cluster sampling would be the most efficient sampling scheme to use, with each school in the state serving as a cluster. Then, schools would be chosen at random and children sampled at random within each school.

The tables at the end of this chapter are for studies in which a random sample were chosen, so we shall make that assumption. (See the discussion and references in Chapter 8 for estimating sample size for cluster sampling.)

We would like to know how many children to select randomly from the state to estimate accurately the percentage (denoted P) of children with breathing problems. We first must decide how accurately we wish to estimate this percentage. We want to estimate P correctly to within 3%; thus, $B = .03$. Then we must decide how confident we wish to be that the resulting interval established from our data will contain the true value of P. We wish to be very confident, so we choose a confidence coefficient of 99%; thus, $CC = .99$. Finally, we must guess at an approximate value of P. We believe P to be approximately 20%; thus, we choose $P = .20$. From Table 10.1, can you find the sample size required to achieve the research objective by meeting the defined criteria? From row 48, we see that a sample size of 1175 is needed to achieve the research objective. If this sample size is larger than we can afford to obtain, we may reduce CC, thereby reducing our confidence that the resulting confidence interval contains the true value of the parameter. Alternatively, we may increase the bound on the error, thereby creating a larger confidence interval. Either change would allow us a smaller sample size, but also would reduce the accuracy of the estimate or our confidence in the results.

If we were planning on taking a larger sample, we have found out that we need not do so to achieve our objective, or we may decide to strive for a lower bound on error. This change would result in a larger sample size. We probably would not increase our confidence coefficient, because 99% is very large already.

10.4 COMPUTING SAMPLE SIZE FOR ESTIMATING $P_1 - P_2$

Suppose that in this project, our objective were to estimate the difference between the percentages of children residing in urban and in rural areas who have breathing problems. We define:

P_U: The true percentage of urban children having breathing problems

P_R: The true percentage of rural children having breathing problems

Then we are less interested in either individual parameter than we are in their difference; thus, we would like to estimate $P_U - P_R$. To accomplish this aim, we must answer the same questions as when we were estimating P. We decide that we would like to estimate this difference to within 5% with 99% confidence; thus, $B = .05$ and $CC = .99$. Now, we must guess at P_U and P_R, and we believe that they are about $P_U = .25$ and $P_R = .15$. The sample size needed to achieve our objective with these requirements can be found in Table 10.2.

The item P_1 always refers to the smaller parameter value: thus, for this example, $P_1 = .15$. The item P_2 refers to the larger parameter value: thus, $P_2 = .25$. The column labeled CC lists the values for the confidence coefficient, and for this example, $CC = .99$. The remaining columns represent various bounds from .01 to .10, and the numbers in the table reflect the sample sizes required in each of the two groups to achieve the research objective. Thus, for $P_1 = .15$, $P_2 = .25$, $B = .05$, and $CC = .99$, we see from row 153 that $n = 833$. Thus, the researcher must sample 833 children from both the urban and the rural areas to achieve the research objective with the above requirements.

Return to Project 10.1 and assume that the objective now is to estimate the difference in the percentage of generic substitutions made between independent and chain pharmacies. We define

P_C: The true percentage of generic substitutions made in chain pharmacies

P_I: The true percentage of generic substitutions made in independent pharmacies

Now we are interested in estimating $P_C - P_I$. We would like to estimate the difference to within 3% with 95% confidence; thus, $B = .03$ and $CC = .95$. We guess that P_C is about 10% and P_I about 5%; thus, $P_1 = .05$ and $P_2 = .10$.

Table 10.2 Sample sizes required to estimate $P_1 - P_2$ for various confidence coefficients and bounds

				BOUND									
Row	P_1	P_2	*CC*	.01	.02	.03	.04	.05	.06	.07	.08	.09	.10
1	0.01	0.01	0.90	536	134	60	34	22	15	11	9	7	6
2	0.01	0.01	0.95	761	191	85	48	31	22	16	12	10	8
3	0.01	0.01	0.99	1308	327	146	82	53	37	27	21	17	14
4	0.01	0.02	0.90	799	200	89	50	32	23	17	13	10	8
5	0.01	0.02	0.95	1134	284	126	71	46	32	24	18	14	12
6	0.01	0.02	0.99	1949	488	217	122	78	55	40	31	25	20
7	0.01	0.03	0.90	1056	264	118	66	43	30	22	17	14	11
8	0.01	0.03	0.95	1499	375	167	94	60	42	31	24	19	15
9	0.01	0.03	0.99	2576	644	287	161	104	72	53	41	32	26
10	0.01	0.04	0.90	1308	327	146	82	53	37	27	21	17	14
11	0.01	0.04	0.95	1856	464	207	116	75	52	38	29	23	19
12	0.01	0.04	0.99	3191	798	355	200	128	89	66	50	40	32
13	0.01	0.05	0.90	1554	389	173	98	63	44	32	25	20	16
14	0.01	0.05	0.95	2206	552	246	138	89	62	46	35	28	23
15	0.01	0.05	0.99	3792	948	422	237	152	106	78	60	47	38
16	0.01	0.10	0.90	2704	676	301	169	109	76	56	43	34	28
17	0.01	0.10	0.95	3838	960	427	240	154	107	79	60	48	39
18	0.01	0.10	0.99	6599	1650	734	413	264	184	135	104	82	66
19	0.01	0.15	0.90	3719	930	414	233	149	104	76	59	46	38
20	0.01	0.15	0.95	5279	1320	587	330	212	147	108	83	66	53
21	0.01	0.15	0.99	9076	2269	1009	568	364	253	186	142	113	91
22	0.01	0.20	0.90	4598	1150	511	288	184	128	94	72	57	46
23	0.01	0.20	0.95	6527	1632	726	408	262	182	134	102	81	66
24	0.01	0.20	0.99	11222	2806	1247	702	449	312	230	176	139	113
25	0.01	0.25	0.90	5342	1336	594	334	214	149	110	84	66	54
26	0.01	0.25	0.95	7584	1896	843	474	304	211	155	119	94	76
27	0.01	0.25	0.99	13039	3260	1449	815	522	363	267	204	161	131
28	0.01	0.30	0.90	5951	1488	662	372	239	166	122	93	74	60
29	0.01	0.30	0.95	8448	2112	939	528	338	235	173	132	105	85
30	0.01	0.30	0.99	14525	3632	1614	908	581	404	297	227	180	146
31	0.01	0.35	0.90	6425	1607	714	402	257	179	132	101	80	65
32	0.01	0.35	0.95	9120	2280	1014	570	365	254	187	143	113	92
33	0.01	0.35	0.99	15681	3921	1743	981	628	436	321	246	194	157
34	0.01	0.40	0.90	6763	1691	752	423	271	188	139	106	84	68
35	0.01	0.40	0.95	9601	2401	1067	601	385	267	196	151	119	97
36	0.01	0.40	0.99	16506	4127	1834	1032	661	459	337	258	204	166
37	0.01	0.45	0.90	6966	1742	774	436	279	194	143	109	86	70
38	0.01	0.45	0.95	9889	2473	1099	619	396	275	202	155	123	99
39	0.01	0.45	0.99	17002	4251	1890	1063	681	473	347	266	210	171
40	0.01	0.50	0.90	7033	1759	782	440	282	196	144	110	87	71
41	0.01	0.50	0.95	9985	2497	1110	625	400	278	204	157	124	100
42	0.01	0.50	0.99	17167	4292	1908	1073	687	477	351	269	212	172
43	0.05	0.05	0.90	2571	643	286	161	103	72	53	41	32	26
44	0.05	0.05	0.95	3650	913	406	229	146	102	75	58	46	37
45	0.05	0.05	0.99	6275	1569	698	393	251	175	129	99	78	63
46	0.05	0.06	0.90	2812	703	313	176	113	79	58	44	35	29
47	0.05	0.06	0.95	3992	998	444	250	160	111	82	63	50	40
48	0.05	0.06	0.99	6863	1716	763	429	275	191	141	108	85	69
49	0.05	0.07	0.90	3047	762	339	191	122	85	63	48	38	31
50	0.05	0.07	0.95	4326	1082	481	271	174	121	89	68	54	44
51	0.05	0.07	0.99	7438	1860	827	465	298	207	152	117	92	75
52	0.05	0.08	0.90	3277	820	365	205	132	92	67	52	41	33
53	0.05	0.08	0.95	4653	1164	517	291	187	130	95	73	58	47
54	0.05	0.08	0.99	7999	2000	889	500	320	223	164	125	99	80
55	0.05	0.09	0.90	3502	876	390	219	141	98	72	55	44	36
56	0.05	0.09	0.95	4972	1243	553	311	199	139	102	78	62	50
57	0.05	0.09	0.99	8547	2137	950	535	342	238	175	134	106	86
58	0.05	0.10	0.90	3721	931	414	233	149	104	76	59	46	38
59	0.05	0.10	0.95	5283	1321	587	331	212	147	108	83	66	53
60	0.05	0.10	0.99	9082	2271	1010	568	364	253	186	142	113	91
61	0.05	0.15	0.90	4736	1184	527	296	190	132	97	74	59	48
62	0.05	0.15	0.95	6723	1681	747	421	269	187	138	106	83	68
63	0.05	0.15	0.99	11559	2890	1285	723	463	322	236	181	143	116
64	0.05	0.20	0.90	5616	1404	624	351	225	156	115	88	70	57
65	0.05	0.20	0.95	7972	1993	886	499	319	222	163	125	99	80
66	0.05	0.20	0.99	13706	3427	1523	857	549	381	280	215	170	138
67	0.05	0.25	0.90	6360	1590	707	398	255	177	130	100	79	64
68	0.05	0.25	0.95	9028	2257	1004	565	362	251	185	142	112	91
69	0.05	0.25	0.99	15522	3881	1725	971	621	432	317	243	192	156
70	0.05	0.30	0.90	6969	1743	775	436	279	194	143	109	87	70
71	0.05	0.30	0.95	9893	2474	1100	619	396	275	202	155	123	99
72	0.05	0.30	0.99	17008	4252	1890	1063	681	473	348	266	210	171
73	0.05	0.35	0.90	7442	1861	827	466	298	207	152	117	92	75
74	0.05	0.35	0.95	10565	2642	1174	661	423	294	216	166	131	106
75	0.05	0.35	0.99	18164	4541	2019	1136	727	505	371	284	225	182

Table 10.2 (continued)

Row	P_1	P_2	CC	BOUND .01	.02	.03	.04	.05	.06	.07	.08	.09	.10
76	0.05	0.40	0.90	7780	1945	865	487	312	217	159	122	97	78
77	0.05	0.40	0.95	11045	2762	1228	691	442	307	226	173	137	111
78	0.05	0.40	0.99	18990	4748	2110	1187	760	528	388	297	235	190
79	0.05	0.45	0.90	7983	1996	887	499	320	222	163	125	99	80
80	0.05	0.45	0.95	11333	2834	1260	709	454	315	232	178	140	114
81	0.05	0.45	0.99	19485	4872	2165	1218	780	542	398	305	241	195
82	0.05	0.50	0.90	8051	2013	895	504	323	224	165	126	100	81
83	0.05	0.50	0.95	11429	2858	1270	715	458	318	234	179	142	115
84	0.05	0.50	0.99	19650	4913	2184	1229	786	546	402	308	243	197
85	0.05	0.55	0.90	7983	1996	887	499	320	222	163	125	99	80
86	0.05	0.55	0.95	11333	2834	1260	709	454	315	232	178	140	114
87	0.05	0.55	0.99	19485	4872	2165	1218	780	542	398	305	241	195
88	0.10	0.10	0.90	4871	1218	542	305	195	136	100	77	61	49
89	0.10	0.10	0.95	6915	1729	769	433	277	193	142	109	86	70
90	0.10	0.10	0.99	11889	2973	1321	744	476	331	243	186	147	119
91	0.10	0.11	0.90	5085	1272	565	318	204	142	104	80	63	51
92	0.10	0.11	0.95	7219	1805	803	452	289	201	148	113	90	73
93	0.10	0.11	0.99	12411	3103	1379	776	497	345	254	194	154	125
94	0.10	0.12	0.90	5293	1324	589	331	212	148	109	83	65	53
95	0.10	0.12	0.95	7515	1879	835	470	301	209	154	118	93	76
96	0.10	0.12	0.99	12920	3230	1436	808	517	359	264	202	160	130
97	0.10	0.13	0.90	5496	1374	611	344	220	153	113	86	68	55
98	0.10	0.13	0.95	7803	1951	867	488	313	217	160	122	97	79
99	0.10	0.13	0.99	13415	3354	1491	839	537	373	274	210	166	135
100	0.10	0.14	0.90	5694	1424	633	356	228	159	117	89	71	57
101	0.10	0.14	0.95	8083	2021	899	506	324	225	165	127	100	81
102	0.10	0.14	0.99	13897	3475	1545	869	556	387	284	218	172	139
103	0.10	0.15	0.90	5886	1472	654	368	236	164	121	92	73	59
104	0.10	0.15	0.95	8356	2089	929	523	335	233	171	131	104	84
105	0.10	0.15	0.99	14366	3592	1597	898	575	400	294	225	178	144
106	0.10	0.20	0.90	6766	1692	752	423	271	188	139	106	84	68
107	0.10	0.20	0.95	9604	2402	1068	601	385	267	197	151	119	97
108	0.10	0.20	0.99	16513	4129	1835	1033	661	459	337	259	204	166
109	0.10	0.25	0.90	7510	1878	835	470	301	209	154	118	93	76
110	0.10	0.25	0.95	10661	2666	1185	667	427	297	218	167	132	107
111	0.10	0.25	0.99	18329	4583	2037	1146	734	510	375	287	227	184
112	0.10	0.30	0.90	8119	2030	903	508	325	226	166	127	101	82
113	0.10	0.30	0.95	11525	2882	1281	721	461	321	236	181	143	116
114	0.10	0.30	0.99	19815	4954	2202	1239	793	551	405	310	245	199
115	0.10	0.35	0.90	8592	2148	955	537	344	239	176	135	107	86
116	0.10	0.35	0.95	12198	3050	1356	763	488	339	249	191	151	122
117	0.10	0.35	0.99	20971	5243	2331	1311	839	583	428	328	259	210
118	0.10	0.40	0.90	8930	2233	993	559	358	249	183	140	111	90
119	0.10	0.40	0.95	12678	3170	1409	793	508	353	259	199	157	127
120	0.10	0.40	0.99	21797	5450	2422	1363	872	606	445	341	270	218
121	0.10	0.45	0.90	9133	2284	1015	571	366	254	187	143	113	92
122	0.10	0.45	0.95	12966	3242	1441	811	519	361	265	203	161	130
123	0.10	0.45	0.99	22292	5573	2477	1394	892	620	455	349	276	223
124	0.10	0.50	0.90	9201	2301	1023	576	369	256	188	144	114	93
125	0.10	0.50	0.95	13062	3266	1452	817	523	363	267	205	162	131
126	0.10	0.50	0.99	22457	5615	2496	1404	899	624	459	351	278	225
127	0.10	0.55	0.90	9133	2284	1015	571	366	254	187	143	113	92
128	0.10	0.55	0.95	12966	3242	1441	811	519	361	265	203	161	130
129	0.10	0.55	0.99	22292	5573	2477	1394	892	620	455	349	276	223
130	0.10	0.60	0.90	8930	2233	993	559	358	249	183	140	111	90
131	0.10	0.60	0.95	12678	3170	1409	793	508	353	259	199	157	127
132	0.10	0.60	0.99	21797	5450	2422	1363	872	606	445	341	270	218
133	0.15	0.15	0.90	6901	1726	767	432	277	192	141	108	86	70
134	0.15	0.15	0.95	9797	2450	1089	613	392	273	200	154	121	98
135	0.15	0.15	0.99	16843	4211	1872	1053	674	468	344	264	208	169
136	0.15	0.16	0.90	7088	1772	788	443	284	197	145	111	88	71
137	0.15	0.16	0.95	10062	2516	1118	629	403	280	206	158	125	101
138	0.15	0.16	0.99	17299	4325	1923	1082	692	481	354	271	214	173
139	0.15	0.17	0.90	7269	1818	808	455	291	202	149	114	90	73
140	0.15	0.17	0.95	10319	2580	1147	645	413	287	211	162	128	104
141	0.15	0.17	0.99	17741	4436	1972	1109	710	493	363	278	220	178
142	0.15	0.18	0.90	7445	1862	828	466	298	207	152	117	92	75
143	0.15	0.18	0.95	10569	2643	1175	661	423	294	216	166	131	106
144	0.15	0.18	0.99	18171	4543	2019	1136	727	505	371	284	225	182
145	0.15	0.19	0.90	7615	1904	847	476	305	212	156	119	95	77
146	0.15	0.19	0.95	10811	2703	1202	676	433	301	221	169	134	109
147	0.15	0.19	0.99	18587	4647	2066	1162	744	517	380	291	230	186
148	0.15	0.20	0.90	7780	1945	865	487	312	217	159	122	97	78
149	0.15	0.20	0.95	11045	2762	1228	691	442	307	226	173	137	111
150	0.15	0.20	0.99	18990	4748	2110	1187	760	528	388	297	235	190

Table 10.2 (*continued*)

Row	P_1	P_2	CC	BOUND .01	.02	.03	.04	.05	.06	.07	.08	.09	.10
151	0.15	0.25	0.90	8524	2131	948	533	341	237	174	134	106	86
152	0.15	0.25	0.95	12102	3026	1345	757	485	337	247	190	150	122
153	0.15	0.25	0.99	20806	5202	2312	1301	833	578	425	326	257	209
154	0.15	0.30	0.90	9133	2284	1015	571	366	254	187	143	113	92
155	0.15	0.30	0.95	12966	3242	1441	811	519	361	265	203	161	130
156	0.15	0.30	0.99	22292	5573	2477	1394	892	620	455	349	276	223
157	0.15	0.35	0.90	9607	2402	1068	601	385	267	197	151	119	97
158	0.15	0.35	0.95	13638	3410	1516	853	546	379	279	214	169	137
159	0.15	0.35	0.99	23448	5862	2606	1466	938	652	479	367	290	235
160	0.15	0.40	0.90	9945	2487	1105	622	398	277	203	156	123	100
161	0.15	0.40	0.95	14118	3530	1569	883	565	393	289	221	175	142
162	0.15	0.40	0.99	24274	6069	2698	1518	971	675	496	380	300	243
163	0.15	0.45	0.90	10148	2537	1128	635	406	282	208	159	126	102
164	0.15	0.45	0.95	14406	3602	1601	901	577	401	295	226	178	145
165	0.15	0.45	0.99	24769	6193	2753	1549	991	689	506	388	306	248
166	0.15	0.50	0.90	10216	2554	1136	639	409	284	209	160	127	103
167	0.15	0.50	0.95	14503	3626	1612	907	581	403	296	227	180	146
168	0.15	0.50	0.99	24934	6234	2771	1559	998	693	509	390	308	250
169	0.15	0.55	0.90	10148	2537	1128	635	406	282	208	159	126	102
170	0.15	0.55	0.95	14406	3602	1601	901	577	401	295	226	178	145
171	0.15	0.55	0.99	24769	6193	2753	1549	991	689	506	388	306	248
172	0.15	0.60	0.90	9945	2487	1105	622	398	277	203	156	123	100
173	0.15	0.60	0.95	14118	3530	1569	883	565	393	289	221	175	142
174	0.15	0.60	0.99	24274	6069	2698	1518	971	675	496	380	300	243
175	0.15	0.65	0.90	9607	2402	1068	601	385	267	197	151	119	97
176	0.15	0.65	0.95	13638	3410	1516	853	546	379	279	214	169	137
177	0.15	0.65	0.99	23448	5862	2606	1466	938	652	479	367	290	235
178	0.20	0.20	0.90	8660	2165	963	542	347	241	177	136	107	87
179	0.20	0.20	0.95	12294	3074	1366	769	492	342	251	193	152	123
180	0.20	0.20	0.99	21136	5284	2349	1321	846	588	432	331	261	212
181	0.20	0.21	0.90	8819	2205	980	552	353	245	180	138	109	89
182	0.20	0.21	0.95	12520	3130	1392	783	501	348	256	196	155	126
183	0.20	0.21	0.99	21526	5382	2392	1346	862	598	440	337	266	216
184	0.20	0.22	0.90	8974	2244	998	561	359	250	184	141	111	90
185	0.20	0.22	0.95	12739	3185	1416	797	510	354	260	200	158	128
186	0.20	0.22	0.99	21902	5476	2434	1369	877	609	447	343	271	220
187	0.20	0.23	0.90	9123	2281	1014	571	365	254	187	143	113	92
188	0.20	0.23	0.95	12951	3238	1439	810	519	360	265	203	160	130
189	0.20	0.23	0.99	22266	5567	2474	1392	891	619	455	348	275	223
190	0.20	0.24	0.90	9266	2317	1030	580	371	258	190	145	115	93
191	0.20	0.24	0.95	13154	3289	1462	823	527	366	269	206	163	132
192	0.20	0.24	0.99	22616	5654	2513	1414	905	629	462	354	280	227
193	0.20	0.25	0.90	9404	2351	1045	588	377	262	192	147	117	95
194	0.20	0.25	0.95	13350	3338	1484	835	534	371	273	209	165	134
195	0.20	0.25	0.99	22953	5739	2551	1435	919	638	469	359	284	230
196	0.20	0.30	0.90	10013	2504	1113	626	401	279	205	157	124	101
197	0.20	0.30	0.95	14214	3554	1580	889	569	395	291	223	176	143
198	0.20	0.30	0.99	24439	6110	2716	1528	978	679	499	382	302	245
199	0.20	0.35	0.90	10486	2622	1166	656	420	292	214	164	130	105
200	0.20	0.35	0.95	14887	3722	1655	931	596	414	304	233	184	149
201	0.20	0.35	0.99	25594	6399	2844	1600	1024	711	523	400	316	256
202	0.20	0.40	0.90	10825	2707	1203	677	433	301	221	170	134	109
203	0.20	0.40	0.95	15367	3842	1708	961	615	427	314	241	190	154
204	0.20	0.40	0.99	26420	6605	2936	1652	1057	734	540	413	327	265
205	0.20	0.45	0.90	11028	2757	1226	690	442	307	226	173	137	111
206	0.20	0.45	0.95	15655	3914	1740	979	627	435	320	245	194	157
207	0.20	0.45	0.99	26915	6729	2991	1683	1077	748	550	421	333	270
208	0.20	0.50	0.90	11095	2774	1233	694	444	309	227	174	137	111
209	0.20	0.50	0.95	15751	3938	1751	985	631	438	322	247	195	158
210	0.20	0.50	0.99	27081	6771	3009	1693	1084	753	553	424	335	271
211	0.20	0.55	0.90	11028	2757	1226	690	442	307	226	173	137	111
212	0.20	0.55	0.95	15655	3914	1740	979	627	435	320	245	194	157
213	0.20	0.55	0.99	26915	6729	2991	1683	1077	748	550	421	333	270
214	0.20	0.60	0.90	10825	2707	1203	677	433	301	221	170	134	109
215	0.20	0.60	0.95	15367	3842	1708	961	615	427	314	241	190	154
216	0.20	0.60	0.99	26420	6605	2936	1652	1057	734	540	413	327	265
217	0.20	0.65	0.90	10486	2622	1166	656	420	292	214	164	130	105
218	0.20	0.65	0.95	14887	3722	1655	931	596	414	304	233	184	149
219	0.20	0.65	0.99	25594	6399	2844	1600	1024	711	523	400	316	256
220	0.20	0.70	0.90	10013	2504	1113	626	401	279	205	157	124	101
221	0.20	0.70	0.95	14214	3554	1580	889	569	395	291	223	176	143
222	0.20	0.70	0.99	24439	6110	2716	1528	978	679	499	382	302	245
223	0.25	0.25	0.90	10148	2537	1128	635	406	282	208	159	126	102
224	0.25	0.25	0.95	14406	3602	1601	901	577	401	295	226	178	145
225	0.25	0.25	0.99	24769	6193	2753	1549	991	689	506	388	306	248

Table 10.2 (*continued*)

				BOUND									
Row	P_1	P_2	*CC*	.01	.02	.03	.04	.05	.06	.07	.08	.09	.10
226	0.25	0.26	0.90	10281	2571	1143	543	412	286	210	161	127	103
227	0.25	0.26	0.95	14595	3649	1622	913	584	406	298	229	181	146
228	0.25	0.26	0.99	25093	6274	2789	1569	1004	698	513	393	310	251
229	0.25	0.27	0.90	10408	2602	1157	651	417	290	213	163	129	105
230	0.25	0.27	0.95	14775	3694	1642	924	591	411	302	231	183	148
231	0.25	0.27	0.99	25403	6351	2823	1588	1017	706	519	397	314	255
232	0.25	0.28	0.90	10530	2633	1170	659	422	293	215	165	130	106
233	0.25	0.28	0.95	14948	3737	1661	935	598	416	306	234	185	150
234	0.25	0.28	0.99	25700	6425	2856	1607	1028	714	525	402	318	257
235	0.25	0.29	0.90	10646	2662	1183	666	426	296	218	167	132	107
236	0.25	0.29	0.95	15113	3779	1680	945	605	420	309	237	187	152
237	0.25	0.29	0.99	25984	6496	2888	1624	1040	722	531	406	321	260
238	0.25	0.30	0.90	10757	2690	1196	673	431	299	220	169	133	108
239	0.25	0.30	0.95	15271	3818	1697	955	611	425	312	239	189	153
240	0.25	0.30	0.99	26255	6564	2918	1641	1051	730	536	411	325	263
241	0.25	0.35	0.90	11231	2808	1248	702	450	312	230	176	139	113
242	0.25	0.35	0.95	15943	3986	1772	997	638	443	326	250	197	160
243	0.25	0.35	0.99	27411	6853	3046	1714	1097	762	560	429	339	275
244	0.25	0.40	0.90	11569	2893	1286	724	463	322	237	181	143	116
245	0.25	0.40	0.95	16423	4106	1825	1027	657	457	336	257	203	165
246	0.25	0.40	0.99	28236	7059	3138	1765	1130	785	577	442	349	283
247	0.25	0.45	0.90	11772	2943	1308	736	471	327	241	184	146	118
248	0.25	0.45	0.95	16711	4178	1857	1045	669	465	342	262	207	168
249	0.25	0.45	0.99	28732	7183	3193	1796	1150	799	587	449	355	288
250	0.25	0.50	0.90	11839	2960	1316	740	474	329	242	185	147	119
251	0.25	0.50	0.95	16807	4202	1868	1051	673	467	344	263	208	169
252	0.25	0.50	0.99	28897	7225	3211	1807	1156	803	590	452	357	289
253	0.25	0.55	0.90	11772	2943	1308	736	471	327	241	184	146	118
254	0.25	0.55	0.95	16711	4178	1857	1045	669	465	342	262	207	168
255	0.25	0.55	0.99	28732	7183	3193	1796	1150	799	587	449	355	288
256	0.25	0.60	0.90	11569	2893	1286	724	463	322	237	181	143	116
257	0.25	0.60	0.95	16423	4106	1825	1027	657	457	336	257	203	165
258	0.25	0.60	0.99	28236	7059	3138	1765	1130	785	577	442	349	283
259	0.25	0.65	0.90	11231	2808	1248	702	450	312	230	176	139	113
260	0.25	0.65	0.95	15943	3986	1772	997	638	443	326	250	197	160
261	0.25	0.65	0.99	27411	6853	3046	1714	1097	762	560	429	339	275
262	0.25	0.70	0.90	10757	2690	1196	673	431	299	220	169	133	108
263	0.25	0.70	0.95	15271	3818	1697	955	611	425	312	239	189	153
264	0.25	0.70	0.99	26255	6564	2918	1641	1051	730	536	411	325	263
265	0.25	0.75	0.90	10148	2537	1128	635	406	282	208	159	126	102
266	0.25	0.75	0.95	14407	3602	1601	901	577	401	295	226	178	145
267	0.25	0.75	0.99	24769	6193	2753	1549	991	689	506	388	306	248
268	0.30	0.30	0.90	11366	2842	1263	711	455	316	232	178	141	114
269	0.30	0.30	0.95	16135	4034	1793	1009	646	449	330	253	200	162
270	0.30	0.30	0.99	27741	6936	3083	1734	1110	771	567	434	343	278
271	0.30	0.31	0.90	11471	2868	1275	717	459	319	235	180	142	115
272	0.30	0.31	0.95	16285	4072	1810	1018	652	453	333	255	202	163
273	0.30	0.31	0.99	27999	7000	3111	1750	1120	778	572	438	346	280
274	0.30	0.32	0.90	11571	2893	1286	724	463	322	237	181	143	116
275	0.30	0.32	0.95	16427	4107	1826	1027	658	457	336	257	203	165
276	0.30	0.32	0.99	28243	7061	3139	1766	1130	785	577	442	349	283
277	0.30	0.33	0.90	11666	2917	1297	730	467	325	239	183	145	117
278	0.30	0.33	0.95	16562	4141	1841	1036	663	461	338	259	205	166
279	0.30	0.33	0.99	28474	7119	3164	1780	1139	791	582	445	352	285
280	0.30	0.34	0.90	11755	2939	1307	735	471	327	240	184	146	118
281	0.30	0.34	0.95	16688	4172	1855	1043	668	464	341	261	207	167
282	0.30	0.34	0.99	28692	7173	3188	1794	1148	797	586	449	355	287
283	0.30	0.35	0.90	11839	2960	1316	740	474	329	242	185	147	119
284	0.30	0.35	0.95	16807	4202	1868	1051	673	467	344	263	208	169
285	0.30	0.35	0.99	28897	7225	3211	1807	1156	803	590	452	357	289
286	0.30	0.40	0.90	12178	3045	1354	762	488	339	249	191	151	122
287	0.30	0.40	0.95	17288	4322	1921	1081	692	481	353	271	214	173
288	0.30	0.40	0.99	29723	7431	3303	1858	1189	826	607	465	367	298
289	0.30	0.45	0.90	12381	3096	1376	774	496	344	253	194	153	124
290	0.30	0.45	0.95	17576	4394	1953	1099	704	489	359	275	217	176
291	0.30	0.45	0.99	30218	7555	3358	1889	1209	840	617	473	374	303
292	0.30	0.50	0.90	12448	3112	1384	778	498	346	255	195	154	125
293	0.30	0.50	0.95	17672	4418	1964	1105	707	491	361	277	219	177
294	0.30	0.50	0.99	30383	7596	3376	1899	1216	844	621	475	376	304
295	0.30	0.55	0.90	12381	3096	1376	774	496	344	253	194	153	124
296	0.30	0.55	0.95	17576	4394	1953	1099	704	489	359	275	217	176
297	0.30	0.55	0.99	30218	7555	3358	1889	1209	840	617	473	374	303
298	0.30	0.60	0.90	12178	3045	1354	762	488	339	249	191	151	122
299	0.30	0.60	0.95	17288	4322	1921	1081	692	481	353	271	214	173
300	0.30	0.60	0.99	29723	7431	3303	1858	1189	826	607	465	367	298

Table 10.2 (*continued*)

Row	P_1	P_2	CC	BOUND .01	.02	.03	.04	.05	.06	.07	.08	.09	.10
301	0.30	0.65	0.90	11839	2960	1316	740	474	329	242	185	147	119
302	0.30	0.65	0.95	16808	4202	1868	1051	673	467	344	263	208	169
303	0.30	0.65	0.99	28897	7225	3211	1807	1156	803	590	452	357	289
304	0.30	0.70	0.90	11366	2842	1263	711	455	316	232	178	141	114
305	0.30	0.70	0.95	16135	4034	1793	1009	646	449	330	253	200	162
306	0.30	0.70	0.99	27741	6936	3083	1734	1110	771	567	434	343	278
307	0.30	0.75	0.90	10757	2690	1196	673	431	299	220	169	133	108
308	0.30	0.75	0.95	15271	3818	1697	955	611	425	312	239	189	153
309	0.30	0.75	0.99	26255	6564	2918	1641	1051	730	536	411	325	263
310	0.30	0.80	0.90	10013	2504	1113	626	401	279	205	157	124	101
311	0.30	0.80	0.95	14214	3554	1580	889	569	395	291	223	176	143
312	0.30	0.80	0.99	24439	6110	2716	1528	978	679	499	382	302	245
313	0.35	0.35	0.90	12313	3079	1369	770	493	343	252	193	153	124
314	0.35	0.35	0.95	17480	4370	1943	1093	700	486	357	274	216	175
315	0.35	0.35	0.99	30053	7514	3340	1879	1203	835	614	470	372	301
316	0.35	0.36	0.90	12391	3098	1377	775	496	345	253	194	153	124
317	0.35	0.36	0.95	17591	4398	1955	1100	704	489	359	275	218	176
318	0.35	0.36	0.99	30244	7561	3361	1891	1210	841	618	473	374	303
319	0.35	0.37	0.90	12464	3116	1385	779	499	347	255	195	154	125
320	0.35	0.37	0.95	17695	4424	1967	1106	708	492	362	277	219	177
321	0.35	0.37	0.99	30423	7606	3381	1902	1217	846	621	476	376	305
322	0.35	0.38	0.90	12532	3133	1393	784	502	349	256	196	155	126
323	0.35	0.38	0.95	17791	4448	1977	1112	712	495	364	278	220	178
324	0.35	0.38	0.99	30588	7647	3399	1912	1224	850	625	478	378	306
325	0.35	0.39	0.90	12594	3149	1400	788	504	350	258	197	156	126
326	0.35	0.39	0.95	17879	4470	1987	1118	716	497	365	280	221	179
327	0.35	0.39	0.99	30740	7685	3416	1922	1230	854	628	481	380	308
328	0.35	0.40	0.90	12651	3163	1406	791	507	352	259	198	157	127
329	0.35	0.40	0.95	17960	4490	1996	1123	719	499	367	281	222	180
330	0.35	0.40	0.99	30878	7720	3431	1930	1236	858	631	483	382	309
331	0.35	0.45	0.90	12854	3214	1429	804	515	358	263	201	159	129
332	0.35	0.45	0.95	18248	4562	2028	1141	730	507	373	286	226	183
333	0.35	0.45	0.99	31374	7844	3486	1961	1255	872	641	491	388	314
334	0.35	0.50	0.90	12922	3231	1436	808	517	359	264	202	160	130
335	0.35	0.50	0.95	18344	4586	2039	1147	734	510	375	287	227	184
336	0.35	0.50	0.99	31539	7885	3505	1972	1262	877	644	493	390	316
337	0.35	0.55	0.90	12854	3214	1429	804	515	358	263	201	159	129
338	0.35	0.55	0.95	18248	4562	2028	1141	730	507	373	286	226	183
339	0.35	0.55	0.99	31374	7844	3486	1961	1255	872	641	491	388	314
340	0.35	0.60	0.90	12651	3163	1406	791	507	352	259	198	157	127
341	0.35	0.60	0.95	17960	4490	1996	1123	719	499	367	281	222	180
342	0.35	0.60	0.99	30878	7720	3431	1930	1236	858	631	483	382	309
343	0.35	0.65	0.90	12313	3079	1369	770	493	343	252	193	153	124
344	0.35	0.65	0.95	17480	4370	1943	1093	700	486	357	274	216	175
345	0.35	0.65	0.99	30053	7514	3340	1879	1203	835	614	470	372	301
346	0.35	0.70	0.90	11839	2960	1316	740	474	329	242	185	147	119
347	0.35	0.70	0.95	16808	4202	1868	1051	673	467	344	263	208	169
348	0.35	0.70	0.99	28897	7225	3211	1807	1156	803	590	452	357	289
349	0.35	0.75	0.90	11231	2808	1248	702	450	312	230	176	139	113
350	0.35	0.75	0.95	15943	3986	1772	997	638	443	326	250	197	160
351	0.35	0.75	0.99	27411	6853	3046	1714	1097	762	560	429	339	275
352	0.35	0.80	0.90	10486	2622	1166	656	420	292	214	164	130	105
353	0.35	0.80	0.95	14887	3722	1655	931	596	414	304	233	184	149
354	0.35	0.80	0.99	25594	6399	2844	1600	1024	711	523	400	316	256
355	0.35	0.85	0.90	9607	2402	1068	601	385	267	197	151	119	97
356	0.35	0.85	0.95	13638	3410	1516	853	546	379	279	214	169	137
357	0.35	0.85	0.99	23448	5862	2606	1466	938	652	479	367	290	235
358	0.40	0.40	0.90	12989	3248	1444	812	520	361	266	203	161	130
359	0.40	0.40	0.95	18440	4610	2049	1153	738	513	377	289	228	185
360	0.40	0.40	0.99	31704	7926	3523	1982	1269	881	648	496	392	318
361	0.40	0.41	0.90	13041	3261	1449	816	522	363	267	204	161	131
362	0.40	0.41	0.95	18513	4629	2057	1158	741	515	378	290	229	186
363	0.40	0.41	0.99	31830	7958	3537	1990	1274	885	650	498	393	319
364	0.40	0.42	0.90	13087	3272	1455	818	524	364	268	205	162	131
365	0.40	0.42	0.95	18578	4645	2065	1162	744	517	380	291	230	186
366	0.40	0.42	0.99	31942	7986	3550	1997	1278	888	652	500	395	320
367	0.40	0.43	0.90	13127	3282	1459	821	526	365	268	206	163	132
368	0.40	0.43	0.95	18636	4659	2071	1165	745	518	381	292	231	187
369	0.40	0.43	0.99	32041	8011	3561	2003	1282	891	654	501	396	321
370	0.40	0.44	0.90	13163	3291	1463	823	527	366	269	206	163	132
371	0.40	0.44	0.95	18686	4672	2077	1168	748	520	382	292	231	187
372	0.40	0.44	0.99	32127	8032	3570	2008	1286	893	656	502	397	322
373	0.40	0.45	0.90	13192	3298	1466	825	528	367	270	207	163	132
374	0.40	0.45	0.95	18728	4682	2081	1171	750	521	383	293	232	188
375	0.40	0.45	0.99	32199	8050	3578	2013	1288	895	658	504	398	322

Table 10.2 (*continued*)

				BOUND									
Row	P_1	P_2	*CC*	.01	.02	.03	.04	.05	.06	.07	.08	.09	.10
376	0.40	0.50	0.90	13260	3315	1474	829	531	369	271	208	164	133
377	0.40	0.50	0.95	18824	4706	2092	1177	753	523	385	295	233	189
378	0.40	0.50	0.99	32365	8092	3597	2023	1295	900	661	506	400	324
379	0.40	0.55	0.90	13192	3298	1466	825	528	367	270	207	163	132
380	0.40	0.55	0.95	18728	4682	2081	1171	750	521	383	293	232	188
381	0.40	0.55	0.99	32199	8050	3578	2013	1288	895	658	504	398	322
382	0.40	0.60	0.90	12989	3248	1444	812	520	361	266	203	151	130
383	0.40	0.60	0.95	18440	4610	2049	1153	738	513	377	289	228	185
384	0.40	0.60	0.99	31704	7926	3523	1982	1269	881	648	496	392	318
385	0.40	0.65	0.90	12651	3163	1406	791	507	352	259	198	157	127
386	0.40	0.65	0.95	17960	4490	1996	1123	719	499	367	281	222	180
387	0.40	0.65	0.99	30878	7720	3431	1930	1236	858	631	483	382	309
388	0.40	0.70	0.90	12178	3045	1354	762	488	339	249	191	151	122
389	0.40	0.70	0.95	17288	4322	1921	1081	692	481	353	271	214	173
390	0.40	0.70	0.99	29723	7431	3303	1858	1189	826	607	465	367	298
391	0.40	0.75	0.90	11569	2893	1286	724	463	322	237	181	143	116
392	0.40	0.75	0.95	16423	4106	1825	1027	657	457	336	257	203	165
393	0.40	0.75	0.99	28236	7059	3138	1765	1130	785	577	442	349	283
394	0.40	0.80	0.90	10825	2707	1203	677	433	301	221	170	134	109
395	0.40	0.80	0.95	15367	3842	1708	961	615	427	314	241	190	154
396	0.40	0.80	0.99	26420	6605	2936	1652	1057	734	540	413	327	265
397	0.40	0.85	0.90	9945	2487	1105	622	398	277	203	156	123	100
398	0.40	0.85	0.95	14118	3530	1569	883	565	393	289	221	175	142
399	0.40	0.85	0.99	24274	6069	2698	1518	971	675	496	380	300	243
400	0.40	0.90	0.90	8930	2233	993	559	358	249	183	140	111	90
401	0.40	0.90	0.95	12678	3170	1409	793	508	353	259	199	157	127
402	0.40	0.90	0.99	21797	5450	2422	1363	872	606	445	341	270	218
403	0.45	0.45	0.90	13395	3349	1489	838	536	373	274	210	166	134
404	0.45	0.45	0.95	19016	4754	2113	1189	761	529	389	298	235	191
405	0.45	0.45	0.99	32695	8174	3633	2044	1308	909	668	511	404	327
406	0.45	0.46	0.90	13420	3355	1492	839	537	373	274	210	166	135
407	0.45	0.46	0.95	19051	4763	2117	1191	763	530	389	298	236	191
408	0.45	0.46	0.99	32754	8189	3640	2048	1311	910	669	512	405	328
409	0.45	0.47	0.90	13439	3360	1494	840	538	374	275	210	166	135
410	0.45	0.47	0.95	19078	4770	2120	1193	764	530	390	299	236	191
411	0.45	0.47	0.99	32800	8200	3645	2050	1312	912	670	513	405	328
412	0.45	0.48	0.90	13452	3363	1495	841	539	374	275	211	167	135
413	0.45	0.48	0.95	19097	4775	2122	1194	764	531	390	299	236	191
414	0.45	0.48	0.99	32833	8209	3649	2053	1314	913	671	514	406	329
415	0.45	0.49	0.90	13460	3365	1496	842	539	374	275	211	167	135
416	0.45	0.49	0.95	19109	4778	2124	1195	765	531	390	299	236	192
417	0.45	0.49	0.99	32853	8214	3651	2054	1315	913	671	514	406	329
418	0.45	0.50	0.90	13463	3366	1496	842	539	374	275	211	167	135
419	0.45	0.50	0.95	19112	4778	2124	1195	765	531	391	299	236	192
420	0.45	0.50	0.99	32860	8215	3652	2054	1315	913	671	514	406	329
421	0.45	0.55	0.90	13395	3349	1489	838	536	373	274	210	166	134
422	0.45	0.55	0.95	19016	4754	2113	1189	761	529	389	298	235	191
423	0.45	0.55	0.99	32695	8174	3633	2044	1303	909	668	511	404	327
424	0.45	0.60	0.90	13192	3298	1466	825	528	367	270	207	163	132
425	0.45	0.60	0.95	18728	4682	2081	1171	750	521	383	293	232	188
426	0.45	0.60	0.99	32199	8050	3578	2013	1288	895	658	504	398	322
427	0.45	0.65	0.90	12854	3214	1429	804	515	358	263	201	159	129
428	0.45	0.65	0.95	18248	4562	2028	1141	730	507	373	286	226	183
429	0.45	0.65	0.99	31374	7844	3486	1961	1255	872	641	491	388	314
430	0.45	0.70	0.90	12381	3096	1376	774	496	344	253	194	153	124
431	0.45	0.70	0.95	17576	4394	1953	1099	704	489	359	275	217	176
432	0.45	0.70	0.99	30218	7555	3358	1889	1209	840	617	473	374	303
433	0.45	0.75	0.90	11772	2943	1308	736	471	327	241	184	145	118
434	0.45	0.75	0.95	16711	4178	1857	1045	669	465	342	262	207	168
435	0.45	0.75	0.99	28732	7183	3193	1796	1150	799	587	449	355	288
436	0.45	0.80	0.90	11028	2757	1226	690	442	307	226	173	137	111
437	0.45	0.80	0.95	15655	3914	1740	979	627	435	320	245	194	157
438	0.45	0.80	0.99	26915	6729	2991	1683	1077	748	550	421	333	270
439	0.45	0.85	0.90	10148	2537	1128	635	406	282	208	159	126	102
440	0.45	0.85	0.95	14407	3602	1601	901	577	401	295	226	178	145
441	0.45	0.85	0.99	24769	6193	2753	1549	991	689	506	388	306	248
442	0.45	0.90	0.90	9133	2284	1015	571	366	254	187	143	113	92
443	0.45	0.90	0.95	12966	3242	1441	811	519	361	265	203	161	130
444	0.45	0.90	0.99	22292	5573	2477	1394	892	620	455	349	276	223
445	0.45	0.95	0.90	7983	1996	887	499	320	222	163	125	99	80
446	0.45	0.95	0.95	11333	2834	1260	709	454	315	232	178	140	114
447	0.45	0.95	0.99	19485	4872	2165	1218	780	542	398	305	241	195
448	0.50	0.50	0.90	13531	3383	1504	846	542	376	277	212	168	136
449	0.50	0.50	0.95	19209	4803	2135	1201	769	534	393	301	238	193
450	0.50	0.50	0.99	33025	8257	3670	2065	1321	918	674	517	408	331

Table 10.2 (*continued*)

				BOUND									
Row	P_1	P_2	*CC*	.01	.02	.03	.04	.05	.06	.07	.08	.09	.10
451	0.5	0.51	0.90	13528	3382	1504	846	542	376	277	212	168	136
452	0.5	0.51	0.95	19205	4802	2134	1201	769	534	392	301	238	193
453	0.5	0.51	0.99	33018	8255	3669	2064	1321	918	674	516	408	331
454	0.5	0.52	0.90	13520	3380	1503	845	541	376	276	212	167	136
455	0.5	0.52	0.95	19193	4799	2133	1200	768	534	392	300	237	192
456	0.5	0.52	0.99	32999	8250	3667	2063	1320	917	674	516	408	330
457	0.5	0.53	0.90	13506	3377	1501	845	541	376	276	212	167	136
458	0.5	0.53	0.95	19174	4794	2131	1199	767	533	392	300	237	192
459	0.5	0.53	0.99	32966	8242	3663	2061	1319	916	673	516	407	330
460	0.5	0.54	0.90	13487	3372	1499	843	540	375	276	211	167	135
461	0.5	0.54	0.95	19147	4787	2128	1197	766	532	391	300	237	192
462	0.5	0.54	0.99	32919	8230	3658	2058	1317	915	672	515	407	330
463	0.5	0.55	0.90	13463	3366	1496	842	539	374	275	211	167	135
464	0.5	0.55	0.95	19112	4778	2124	1195	765	531	391	299	236	192
465	0.5	0.55	0.99	32860	8215	3652	2054	1315	913	671	514	406	329
466	0.5	0.60	0.90	13260	3315	1474	829	531	369	271	208	164	133
467	0.5	0.60	0.95	18824	4706	2092	1177	753	523	385	295	233	189
468	0.5	0.60	0.99	32365	8092	3597	2023	1295	900	661	506	400	324
469	0.5	0.65	0.90	12922	3231	1436	808	517	359	264	202	160	130
470	0.5	0.65	0.95	18344	4586	2039	1147	734	510	375	287	227	184
471	0.5	0.65	0.99	31539	7885	3505	1972	1262	877	644	493	390	316
472	0.5	0.70	0.90	12448	3112	1384	778	498	346	255	195	154	125
473	0.5	0.70	0.95	17672	4418	1964	1105	707	491	361	277	219	177
474	0.5	0.70	0.99	30383	7596	3376	1899	1216	844	621	475	376	304
475	0.5	0.75	0.90	11839	2960	1316	740	474	329	242	185	147	119
476	0.5	0.75	0.95	16808	4202	1868	1051	673	467	344	263	208	169
477	0.5	0.75	0.99	28897	7225	3211	1807	1156	803	590	452	357	289
478	0.5	0.80	0.90	11095	2774	1233	694	444	309	227	174	137	111
479	0.5	0.80	0.95	15751	3938	1751	985	631	438	322	247	195	158
480	0.5	0.80	0.99	27081	6771	3009	1693	1084	753	553	424	335	271
481	0.5	0.85	0.90	10216	2554	1136	639	409	284	209	160	127	103
482	0.5	0.85	0.95	14503	3626	1612	907	581	403	296	227	180	146
483	0.5	0.85	0.99	24934	6234	2771	1559	998	693	509	390	308	250
484	0.5	0.90	0.90	9201	2301	1023	576	369	256	188	144	114	93
485	0.5	0.90	0.95	13062	3266	1452	817	523	363	267	205	162	131
486	0.5	0.90	0.99	22457	5615	2496	1404	899	624	459	351	278	225
487	0.5	0.95	0.90	8051	2013	895	504	323	224	165	126	100	81
488	0.5	0.95	0.95	11429	2858	1270	715	458	318	234	179	142	115
489	0.5	0.95	0.99	19650	4913	2184	1229	786	546	402	308	243	197
490	0.5	1.00	0.90	6766	1692	752	423	271	188	139	106	84	68
491	0.5	1.00	0.95	9605	2402	1068	601	385	267	197	151	119	97
492	0.5	1.00	0.99	16513	4129	1835	1033	661	459	337	259	204	166

From Table 10.2, we see that to achieve our objective, the number of prescriptions that we must sample from both chain and independent pharmacies is $n = 587$.

As with Table 10.1, Table 10.2 has P_1 only as large as 50%. If both P_1 and P_2 are larger than 50%, subtract them both from 100% and use Table 10.2 to estimate the needed sample size.

If you would like to compute a sample size not given in the table, the equation to use is

$$n = \frac{Z^2[P_1(1 - P_1) + P_2(1 - P_2)]}{B^2} \tag{10.2}$$

where Z is obtained from a table of standard normal values for a chosen confidence coefficient.

10.5 COMPUTING SAMPLE SIZE FOR ESTIMATING THE PARAMETER μ

Project 10.3 A study of factors related to weight loss following gastric partition surgery

Let us simplify Project 3.1 and make the objective **to estimate the average initial weight loss of patients having gastric partition surgery.** We shall not consider at this point the factors that were defined earlier, but instead, we shall bring them in later.

Table 10.3 Sample sizes required to estimate μ for various delta and confidence coefficients

Row	*DELTA*	*CC*	*N*
1	0.050	0.90	1083
2	0.050	0.95	1537
3	0.050	0.99	2642
4	0.075	0.90	482
5	0.075	0.95	683
6	0.075	0.99	1175
7	0.100	0.90	271
8	0.100	0.95	385
9	0.100	0.99	661
10	0.125	0.90	174
11	0.125	0.95	246
12	0.125	0.99	423
13	0.150	0.90	121
14	0.150	0.95	171
15	0.150	0.99	294
16	0.175	0.90	89
17	0.175	0.95	126
18	0.175	0.99	216
19	0.200	0.90	68
20	0.200	0.95	97
21	0.200	0.99	166
22	0.225	0.90	54
23	0.225	0.95	76
24	0.225	0.99	131
25	0.250	0.90	44
26	0.250	0.95	62
27	0.250	0.99	106
28	0.275	0.90	36
29	0.275	0.95	51
30	0.275	0.99	88
31	0.300	0.90	31
32	0.300	0.95	43
33	0.300	0.99	74
34	0.325	0.90	26
35	0.325	0.95	37
36	0.325	0.99	63
37	0.350	0.90	23
38	0.350	0.95	32
39	0.350	0.99	54
40	0.375	0.90	20
41	0.375	0.95	28
42	0.375	0.99	47
43	0.400	0.90	17
44	0.400	0.95	25
45	0.400	0.99	42
46	0.425	0.90	15
47	0.425	0.95	22
48	0.425	0.99	37
49	0.450	0.90	14
50	0.450	0.95	19
51	0.450	0.99	33
52	0.475	0.90	12
53	0.475	0.95	18
54	0.475	0.99	30
55	0.500	0.90	11
56	0.500	0.95	16
57	0.500	0.99	27

The response variable is the weight loss in the first month following gastric partition surgery, and it should be considered continuous. The parameter of interest is μ, the true average weight loss of all patients having gastric partition surgery.

In addition to answering the questions from the previous section, we must estimate the variability in the response variable measurements. If data have been collected previously, that can be used to estimate the standard deviation, σ; otherwise, the range can be used. The smallest weight loss to be expected would be 0 lb, and the largest weight loss is about 40 lb, so the range of measurements is 40 lb ($40 - 0 = 40$). Thus, σ is estimated to be $\sigma \approx \text{range}/4 = 40/4 = 10$ lb.

Next, we must determine how accurately we would like to estimate μ. Would we like to estimate μ correctly to within 10 lb, or 5, or 2, or .5 lb? Let us say that we wish to estimate μ to within 2 lb: that is, $B = 2$. Now, σ and B can be combined to compute DELTA, which is defined as DELTA $= B/\sigma$. Another response variable may have a range and a bound 10 times greater than this response variable, or one-tenth that of this response variable; and each would require the same sample size. Thus, a table of sample sizes is not needed for each possible σ and B, but only for their ratio.

The final choice is the confidence coefficient, and, for this example, we choose 95%, or $CC = .95$. Table 10.3 contains the sample sizes for estimating μ for various DELTA and confidence coefficients. For this example, with DELTA $= B/\sigma = 2/10 = .2$ and $CC = .95$, we see from row 38 that 97 people would be needed to estimate μ to within 2 lb with 95% confidence.

Let us look at another example.

Project 10.4 Evaluation of the influence of SO_2 on breathing

Refer to Project 3.3 and Project 4.2, whose objective is **to determine whether breathing is affected after prolonged breathing of SO_2.** In this project, there are five response variables and three factors of interest, but for now, let us consider only FEV_1 and no factors.

Suppose we wish to estimate the average FEV_1 of people after breathing SO_2. For the adult universe of interest, the range of FEV_1 is estimated to be 1.5 to 5.5 ℓ; thus, the range is 4 ℓ. The quantity σ then is estimated to be $\sigma \approx \text{range}/4 = 4/4 = 1$ ℓ. We decide that we would like to estimate the average FEV_1, μ, to within .3 ℓ with 99% confidence. Thus, DELTA $= B/\sigma = .3/1 = .3$ and $CC = .99$ and, from row 33 of Table 10.3 we see that the approximate number of people needed for this study is 74.

If your particular study requires a sample size estimation for a value of DELTA or CC not given in Table 10.3, the equation to compute n is

$$n = \left(\frac{Z}{\text{DELTA}}\right)^2 \tag{10.3}$$

where Z is obtained from a table of standard normal values for a chosen confidence coefficient. Remember that for $CC = .90$, $Z = 1.645$; for $CC = .95$, $Z = 1.96$; and for $CC = .99$, $Z = 2.57$.

This project really included five different response variables, and we may wish to estimate a confidence interval for each one. Each response variable would have its own σ and B, and we should compute DELTA for each response variable. The sample size then should be computed for the smallest DELTA, because that approach will result in the largest computed sample size and will provide a confidence interval for each response variable that is less than each desired bound.

Another approach, more appropriate and also more complex, is to compute a **multivariate confidence interval,** which is a confidence interval computed simultaneously for all response variables. A discussion of this procedure is beyond the scope of this book, and if you wish to use it, you should consult a professional statistician.

10.6 COMPUTING SAMPLE SIZE FOR ESTIMATING $\mu_1 - \mu_2$

In this situation, we are estimating the average difference in response variable between two factor levels. We must consider two possible designs here: 1) one in which each experimental unit receives only one factor level and 2) a repeated measure design in which each experimental unit receives both factor levels and has the response variable measured under each. Let us first consider the repeated measure design.

10.6.1 Repeated Measure Design

Let us extend the last example, Project 10.4, to estimate the average difference in FEV_1 between people breathing normal room air and people breathing air with SO_2 added. Thus, the parameters of interest are

μ_A:	Average FEV_1 of people breathing normal room air
μ_S:	Average FEV_1 of people breathing room air and SO_2

We are interested in estimating $\mu_A - \mu_S$ (or $\mu_S - \mu_A$), and each person has FEV_1 measured under each of the two breathing conditions. We must begin by estimating the standard deviation of measurements. Because a repeated measure design is used, we really are most interested in the difference between the two measurements made on an individual rather than in the two individual measurements. Thus, if an individual had an FEV_1 of 3.2 ℓ when breathing room air and 2.7 ℓ when breathing air with SO_2, the measurement of interest is .5, the difference between 3.2 and 2.7. We therefore must estimate the standard deviation of these difference scores (denoted as σ_D). The quantity σ_D can be estimated from the range, as we showed earlier. If the range of FEV_1 is 1.5 to 5.5 ℓ under both conditions, the largest possible range of differences is 8, because the smallest difference is $-4(1.5 - 5.5)$ and the largest difference is $+4(5.5 - 1.5)$.

	Air		**SO_2**
Minimum FEV_1	1.5	+4	1.5
Maximum FEV_1	5.5	−4	5.5

Extreme Differences

$$\text{Minimum Air} - \text{Maximum } SO_2 = 1.5 - 5.5 = -4$$
$$\text{Maximum Air} - \text{Minimum } SO_2 = 5.5 - 1.5 = +4$$

The true range probably will be less, because such extreme differences are unlikely to occur in practice. We may feel that the difference in FEV_1 never will be more than 3 ℓ in either direction, and hence we may use 6 as the estimate of the range. Then σ_D can be estimated as

$$\sigma_D \simeq \frac{\text{range}}{4} = \frac{6}{4} = 1.5.$$

Now, we only need to choose the appropriate bound and confidence coefficient. If we wish to estimate the average difference to within .5 ℓ with 95% confidence, we have $B = .5$ and $\text{DELTA} = B/\sigma = .5/1.5 = .33$ and $CC = .95$. In Table 10.3, DELTA = .33 is not given, so using the nearest value of .325, we see from line 35 that $n = 37$. If we use Eq. 10.3, the estimate of n is

$$n = \left(\frac{Z}{\text{DELTA}}\right)^2 = \left(\frac{1.96}{.33}\right)^2 = 35.3 \qquad \text{or} \qquad n = 36$$

Therefore, about 36 people would be needed in this repeated measure design to estimate the average difference in FEV_1 between breathing room air and air with SO_2 to within .5 ℓ with 95% confidence.

Project 10.5 Evaluation of effect of a drug on intraocular pressure of glaucomatous beagles

A researcher would like to determine whether the intraocular pressure (IOP) in glaucomatous beagles drops after they are given Drug A.

Factor:	Type of drug
Level 1:	No drug
Level 2:	Drug A

In this study each dog will have its IOP measured under no drug. It then will receive a single dose of Drug A and have IOP measured at a suitable later time. Thus, this study is an example of a complete repeated measure design, and the objective is to estimate the average difference in IOP between no drug and Drug A in glaucomatous beagles. Define:

μ_N:	Average IOP in glaucomatous beagles receiving no drug
μ_A:	Average IOP in glaucomatous beagles receiving Drug A

We are interested in estimating $\mu_N - \mu_A$. Because this project has a repeated measure design, we must estimate the standard deviation of the difference of measurements on each beagle, σ_D. If we believe the range in IOP under no drug to be 25 to 40 mm Hg and under Drug A to be 25 to 35 mm Hg, the maximum range of differences would be -10 $(25 - 35)$ to 15 $(40 - 25)$ mm Hg. We may feel, however, that, no change in IOP greater than ± 5 mm Hg is likely to occur, and hence, we may define the range for the difference as 10 $[5 - (-5)]$. Thus,

$$\sigma_D \approx \frac{\text{range}}{4} = \frac{10}{4} = 2.5 \text{ mm Hg}$$

We also decide that we would like to estimate the difference between the parameters to within 1 unit with 95% probability. Thus, $B = 1$, DELTA $= B/\sigma_D = 1/2.5 = .4$, and $CC = .95$. From line 44 of Table 10.3, we see that a sample size of about 25 beagles is needed to estimate $\mu_N - \mu_A$ to within 1 unit with 95% confidence.

10.6.2 No Repeated Measures

Suppose that in the previous example, we wished to evaluate the relationship between type of drug given (Drug A versus Drug B) and IOP of glaucomatous beagles. We still have a single factor with two levels, but repeated measures probably are not possible. Instead, each beagle will receive only one drug in the study. The objective still is to estimate the average difference in IOP between these two drugs, denoted $\mu_A - \mu_B$.

We now must estimate the variability among the response variable measurements within each sample. Let us assume that the variability is the same for the measurements obtained under both drugs: that is, $\sigma_A = \sigma_B$. Then the common standard deviation, denoted σ, can be estimated from the range. If we believe that the range of measurements of IOP is 25 to 35 mm Hg, then the range is 10, and

$$\sigma \approx \frac{\text{range}}{4} = \frac{10}{4} = 2.5 \text{ mm Hg}$$

As before, we wish to estimate the difference $\mu_A - \mu_B$ to within 1 unit with 95% confidence. Thus, $B = 1$, DELTA $= 1/2.5 = .4$, and $CC = .95$. We can find the number of beagles needed in each group in Table 10.3 by finding the n for B, DELTA, and CC given above and *doubling* that number. For this example, we see from line 44 of Table 10.3 that $n = 25$. Then, for this project, we can conclude that 50 beagles are needed *in each group* to achieve the research objective.

If you felt that the variability was different in the measurements in each factor level, you could use the following equation to estimate n:

$$n = \frac{Z^2(\sigma_1^2 + \sigma_2^2)}{B^2} \qquad (10.4)$$

In this case, you would have to estimate both σ_1^2 and σ_2^2. The computed sample size still is the number of experimental units needed in each factor level. Note that if we assume $\sigma_1^2 = \sigma_2^2$, as we did earlier, Eq. 10.4 becomes two times Eq. 10.3.

Let us look at one more example. Return to Project 10.4, and let us now evaluate breathing air plus SO_2 on normals (no breathing problems) versus asthmatics. The response variable still is FEV_1, and the single factor of interest is

Factor:	Group
Level 1:	Normal
Level 2:	Asthmatic

Because a person cannot be in both groups, we do not have a repeated measure design. We define

μ_N:	Average FEV_1 of all normal people
μ_A:	Average FEV_1 of all asthmatic people

We would like to estimate $\mu_N - \mu_A$. In Project 10.4, we estimated $\sigma = 1$ ℓ, so we shall stay with that estimate. We would like to estimate $\mu_N - \mu_A$ to within .3 ℓ with 90% confidence. Thus, $B = .3$, DELTA $= B/\sigma = .3/1 = .3$, and $CC = .9$ and, from line 31 of Table 10.3, we see that $n = 31$. Remember that this number is doubled, so we need about 62 normal people and 62 asthmatics to achieve our research objective.

Let us now look at determining the sample size for a hypothesis-testing inference.

10.7 DETERMINATION OF SAMPLE SIZE TO TEST A HYPOTHESIS

A national survey may have shown that the national generic substitution rate is 10%. We would like to determine whether the generic substitution rate in our state, P, is the same as the national average. Thus, we would like to determine whether $P = .10$, and we would test this statement as the null hypothesis.

Alternatively, we may wish to determine whether the generic substitution rates in two neighboring states are the same. If the unknown rates are denoted P_A and P_B, we would like to know if $P_A = P_B$, and this hypothesis would be H_0.

The same considerations must be taken as in the last few sections, except that instead of choosing a confidence coefficient for the interval estimate, you now must choose a suitable p (or α) and β. Remember that these quantities represent the respective probabilities of making a Type I and a Type II error. (These terms were defined in Chapter 9.) You should have a sample size large enough so that these probabilities are satisfactorily small.

Let us now look at some examples of determining sample size for hypothesis testing. We shall use the same examples used in the earlier sections so that you can contrast an estimation inference with a hypothesis-testing inference. Only tests for the parameters $P_1 - P_2$ and $\mu_1 - \mu_2$ will be considered, because they occur most frequently in practice. A similar approach would exist for other parameters, but the mathematical equation to compute n would change.

10.8 TESTING A HYPOTHESIS ABOUT $P_1 - P_2$

Earlier in this chapter, we defined P_C and P_I as the true percentages of generic substitution made in chain and independent pharmacies, respectively. We then showed how to determine the sample size needed to estimate the difference between these parameters. Suppose, instead, that we wanted to determine whether there was a difference in the generic substitution rate between chain and independent pharmacies: that is, does $P_C = P_I$? The null hypothesis to test is $H_0: P_C = P_I$. In this case, assume that we have no idea of which type of pharmacy may have the higher substitution rate and no particular interest in showing a particular direction. Then the alternative hypothesis should be stated as two tailed: that is, $H_a: P_C \neq P_I$. If we were interested only in showing that a particular type of pharmacy had a higher substitution rate, we might perform a one-tail test, either $H_a: P_C > P_I$ or $H_a: P_C < P_I$. For example, if a large chain pharmacy wished to advertise that their stores performed a service for their customers by filling more generic prescriptions than did independent pharmacies, it would like to show $H_a: P_C > P_I$ and would carry out the appropriate one-tail test. The decision to perform a one or two-tail test is made based on the researcher's intuition and research objective. The alternative hypothesis $\mathbf{H_a}$ **should not be determined after observation of the collected data,** as the probabilities α and β will be different from their chosen values in this case.

A one-tail test does have advantages over a two-tail test in that a smaller sample size is required for a chosen significance level, and also, the power of the test is increased (β is decreased). However, you must be careful to make proper use of the one-tail test. See reference 1 for more on one versus two-tail tests. For our example, we shall consider the two-tail alternative $H_a: P_C \neq P_I$.

Next, we must determine how much of a difference between P_C and P_I is meaningful to detect. Is an important difference 10%, 5%, 1%, or .5%? We must choose the important difference, keeping in mind that the smaller the difference we wish to show, the larger the required sample size. Let us choose 3% as an important difference to show. Finally, α and β must be chosen. For this example, we choose $\alpha = .05$ and $\beta = .2$ (thus, power = 80%).

As in the earlier sections on estimation for a nominal response variable, we must guess at the values of P_C and P_1, because these values are included in the computations. Assume them to be 5% and 8%, and then all the information is available to determine the sample size for this hypothesis. Table 10.4 contains the sample sizes for combinations of P_1, P_2, α, and β. For $P_1 = .05$, $P_2 = .08$, $\alpha = .05$, and power = 80%, we see from line 8 and column 7 of Table 10.4 that $n = 1126$: that is, about 1126 prescriptions would have to be sampled from both chain and independent pharmacies to show a 3% difference in generic substitution rates. Had this test been done as a one-sided test, Table 10.4 still would be used, and the only change would be that the one-tail significance levels would be used.

Table 10.4 Sample sizes required to test $H_0: P_1 = P_2$ for various α and power

$P_1 = .05$										
		α		POWER (%)						
Row	P_2	1-Tail	2-Tail	50	60	70	80	90	95	99
1	0.06	0.050	0.10	3010	3942	5093	6633	9097	11449	16595
2	0.06	0.025	0.05	4191	5289	6517	8365	11117	13706	19299
3	0.06	0.005	0.01	7065	8483	10156	12307	15613	18664	25122
4	0.07	0.050	0.10	861	1114	1426	1844	2512	3149	4544
5	0.07	0.025	0.05	1182	1480	1840	2314	3060	3762	5278
6	0.07	0.005	0.01	1962	2346	2800	3383	4280	5107	6857
7	0.08	0.050	0.10	430	551	701	901	1221	1526	2193
8	0.08	0.025	0.05	584	727	899	1126	1483	1819	2544
9	0.08	0.005	0.01	958	1142	1359	1638	2067	2463	3300
10	0.09	0.050	0.10	268	342	432	552	744	928	1329
11	0.09	0.025	0.05	361	447	551	688	902	1105	1541
12	0.09	0.005	0.01	587	698	828	996	1254	1492	1996
13	0.10	0.050	0.10	189	239	300	382	513	638	911
14	0.10	0.025	0.05	252	311	382	475	621	758	1055
15	0.10	0.005	0.01	406	482	571	685	861	1023	1365
16	0.15	0.050	0.10	68	84	104	130	172	212	300
17	0.15	0.025	0.05	89	107	130	160	207	251	346
18	0.15	0.005	0.01	139	163	192	228	285	337	446
19	0.20	0.050	0.10	39	48	58	72	95	116	162
20	0.20	0.025	0.05	50	60	73	89	113	137	187
21	0.20	0.005	0.01	77	90	106	125	155	183	241
22	0.25	0.050	0.10	27	32	39	48	63	76	106
23	0.25	0.025	0.05	34	41	49	59	75	90	122
24	0.25	0.005	0.01	52	61	70	83	102	120	157
25	0.30	0.050	0.10	20	24	29	36	46	55	77
26	0.30	0.025	0.05	26	30	36	43	55	65	88
27	0.30	0.005	0.01	39	45	52	61	74	87	113
28	0.35	0.050	0.10	16	19	23	28	35	43	58
29	0.35	0.025	0.05	20	24	28	34	42	50	67
30	0.35	0.005	0.01	30	35	40	47	57	67	86
31	0.40	0.050	0.10	13	16	19	22	28	34	46
32	0.40	0.025	0.05	17	19	23	27	34	40	53
33	0.40	0.005	0.01	25	28	32	38	46	53	69
34	0.45	0.050	0.10	11	13	16	19	23	28	38
35	0.45	0.025	0.05	14	16	19	22	28	33	43
36	0.45	0.005	0.01	21	24	27	31	38	43	56
37	0.50	0.050	0.10	10	11	13	16	20	23	31
38	0.50	0.025	0.05	12	14	16	19	23	27	36
39	0.50	0.005	0.01	18	20	23	26	31	36	46
40	0.55	0.050	0.10	9	10	11	13	17	20	26
41	0.55	0.025	0.05	11	12	14	16	20	23	30
42	0.55	0.005	0.01	15	17	20	22	27	31	39

Table 10.4 (*continued*)

		$P_1 = .1$								
		α		POWER (%)						
Row	P_2	*1-Tail*	*2-Tail*	50	60	70	80	90	95	99
43	0.11	0.050	0.10	5285	6970	9049	11833	16289	20541	29848
44	0.11	0.025	0.05	7419	9404	11805	14966	19940	24623	34737
45	0.11	0.005	0.01	12614	15178	18203	22092	28071	33588	45266
46	0.12	0.050	0.10	1423	1862	2404	3129	4289	5396	7818
47	0.12	0.025	0.05	1980	2496	3122	3945	5240	6459	9091
48	0.12	0.005	0.01	3333	4001	4788	5801	7357	8793	11833
49	0.13	0.050	0.10	678	880	1131	1465	2001	2512	3630
50	0.13	0.025	0.05	935	1174	1462	1842	2440	3003	4218
51	0.13	0.005	0.01	1560	1869	2232	2700	3418	4082	5485
52	0.14	0.050	0.10	406	525	671	866	1178	1476	2128
53	0.14	0.025	0.05	556	696	864	1086	1435	1763	2471
54	0.14	0.005	0.01	922	1102	1314	1586	2005	2392	3210
55	0.15	0.050	0.10	276	354	451	580	787	984	1416
56	0.15	0.025	0.05	376	468	579	726	957	1174	1643
57	0.15	0.005	0.01	618	737	877	1058	1335	1591	2133
58	0.20	0.050	0.10	88	111	139	177	237	293	418
59	0.20	0.025	0.05	118	144	177	219	286	349	484
60	0.20	0.005	0.01	188	223	264	316	396	470	626
61	0.25	0.050	0.10	48	59	73	92	121	150	211
62	0.25	0.025	0.05	62	76	92	113	146	177	244
63	0.25	0.005	0.01	98	115	136	162	201	238	316
64	0.30	0.050	0.10	31	38	47	59	77	94	132
65	0.30	0.025	0.05	41	49	59	72	92	111	152
66	0.30	0.005	0.01	63	74	86	102	126	149	196
67	0.35	0.050	0.10	23	28	34	42	54	66	92
68	0.35	0.025	0.05	29	35	42	51	65	78	106
69	0.35	0.005	0.01	45	52	61	72	89	104	136
70	0.40	0.050	0.10	18	21	26	32	41	49	68
71	0.40	0.025	0.05	23	27	32	38	49	58	79
72	0.40	0.005	0.01	34	40	46	54	66	78	101
73	0.45	0.050	0.10	14	17	21	25	32	38	53
74	0.45	0.025	0.05	18	21	25	30	38	45	61
75	0.45	0.005	0.01	27	32	36	42	52	60	78
76	0.50	0.050	0.10	12	14	17	20	26	31	42
77	0.50	0.025	0.05	15	18	21	25	31	36	49
78	0.50	0.005	0.01	23	26	30	34	42	48	62
79	0.55	0.050	0.10	10	12	14	17	21	25	34
80	0.55	0.025	0.05	13	15	17	20	25	30	40
81	0.55	0.005	0.01	19	22	25	28	34	40	51
82	0.60	0.050	0.10	9	10	12	14	18	21	28
83	0.60	0.025	0.05	11	13	15	17	21	25	33
84	0.60	0.005	0.01	16	18	21	24	29	33	42

Table 10.4 (*continued*)

$P_1 = .15$

Row	P_2	α 1-Tail	α 2-Tail	POWER (%) 50	60	70	80	90	95	99
85	0.16	0.050	0.10	7288	9636	12534	16414	22625	28551	41523
86	0.16	0.025	0.05	10263	13028	16375	20780	27714	34240	48337
87	0.16	0.005	0.01	17501	21075	25292	30712	39045	46735	63012
88	0.17	0.050	0.10	1918	2520	3264	4259	5852	7371	10698
89	0.17	0.025	0.05	2681	3391	4249	5379	7157	8831	12446
90	0.17	0.005	0.01	4538	5455	6536	7927	10064	12036	16210
91	0.18	0.050	0.10	894	1169	1508	1961	2686	3378	4893
92	0.18	0.025	0.05	1242	1566	1957	2471	3281	4043	5689
93	0.18	0.005	0.01	2089	2506	2999	3632	4605	5503	7403
94	0.19	0.050	0.10	527	685	880	1141	1558	1957	2828
95	0.19	0.025	0.05	727	913	1138	1435	1901	2339	3287
96	0.19	0.005	0.01	1215	1455	1739	2103	2663	3180	4274
97	0.20	0.050	0.10	352	455	583	754	1027	1288	1858
98	0.20	0.025	0.05	483	605	753	946	1251	1538	2158
99	0.20	0.005	0.01	803	960	1146	1384	1751	2089	2804
100	0.25	0.050	0.10	106	135	170	217	292	364	521
101	0.25	0.025	0.05	143	176	217	270	354	433	603
102	0.25	0.005	0.01	231	275	326	392	492	585	782
103	0.30	0.050	0.10	55	69	86	108	144	179	254
104	0.30	0.025	0.05	73	89	108	134	174	212	294
105	0.30	0.005	0.01	116	137	161	193	241	286	380
106	0.35	0.050	0.10	35	43	54	67	89	109	154
107	0.35	0.025	0.05	46	56	67	83	107	129	178
108	0.35	0.005	0.01	72	85	99	118	147	173	229
109	0.40	0.050	0.10	25	31	38	47	61	75	104
110	0.40	0.025	0.05	33	39	47	57	73	88	121
111	0.40	0.005	0.01	50	59	69	81	100	118	156
112	0.45	0.050	0.10	19	23	28	35	45	55	76
113	0.45	0.025	0.05	25	29	35	42	54	65	88
114	0.45	0.005	0.01	38	44	51	60	74	86	113
115	0.50	0.050	0.10	15	18	22	27	35	42	58
116	0.50	0.025	0.05	20	23	27	33	42	50	67
117	0.50	0.005	0.01	30	34	39	46	57	66	86
118	0.55	0.050	0.10	13	15	18	22	28	33	46
119	0.55	0.025	0.05	16	19	22	26	33	39	53
120	0.55	0.005	0.01	24	28	32	37	45	52	68
121	0.60	0.050	0.10	11	13	15	18	23	27	37
122	0.60	0.025	0.05	13	16	18	22	27	32	42
123	0.60	0.005	0.01	20	23	26	30	37	42	54
124	0.65	0.050	0.10	9	11	13	15	19	22	30
125	0.65	0.025	0.05	12	13	15	18	22	26	35
126	0.65	0.005	0.01	17	19	22	25	30	35	45

Table 10.4 (continued)

				$P_1 = .2$						
		α		POWER (%)						
Row	P_2	*1-Tail*	*2-Tail*	50	60	70	80	90	95	99
127	0.21	0.050	0.10	9020	11941	15548	20376	28104	35479	51620
128	0.21	0.025	0.05	12721	16163	20328	25808	34436	42558	60100
129	0.21	0.005	0.01	21729	26176	31422	38167	48537	58106	78359
130	0.22	0.050	0.10	2344	3088	4005	5234	7200	9076	13183
131	0.22	0.025	0.05	3286	4162	5222	6616	8811	10878	15340
132	0.22	0.005	0.01	5579	6710	8045	9761	12399	14834	19987
133	0.23	0.050	0.10	1081	1417	1832	2387	3276	4124	5980
134	0.23	0.025	0.05	1507	1903	2382	3012	4004	4938	6955
135	0.23	0.005	0.01	2544	3055	3659	4434	5627	6727	9055
136	0.24	0.050	0.10	630	822	1059	1377	1885	2369	3430
137	0.24	0.025	0.05	874	1100	1374	1734	2301	2835	3988
138	0.24	0.005	0.01	1467	1759	2104	2547	3229	3858	5189
139	0.25	0.050	0.10	417	542	696	903	1233	1547	2237
140	0.25	0.025	0.05	576	723	901	1135	1503	1850	2599
141	0.25	0.005	0.01	961	1152	1376	1664	2107	2515	3380
142	0.30	0.050	0.10	121	155	196	251	339	423	607
143	0.30	0.025	0.05	164	203	251	314	412	505	705
144	0.30	0.005	0.01	268	319	379	456	574	683	914
145	0.35	0.050	0.10	61	77	96	122	163	203	289
146	0.35	0.025	0.05	81	100	122	152	198	241	334
147	0.35	0.005	0.01	131	154	183	219	274	325	433
148	0.40	0.050	0.10	38	48	59	74	98	121	171
149	0.40	0.025	0.05	50	61	74	92	118	144	198
150	0.40	0.005	0.01	80	94	110	131	164	193	256
151	0.45	0.050	0.10	27	33	41	51	66	82	114
152	0.45	0.025	0.05	35	42	51	62	80	97	132
153	0.45	0.005	0.01	55	64	75	89	110	130	171
154	0.50	0.050	0.10	20	25	30	37	48	59	82
155	0.50	0.025	0.05	26	31	37	45	58	70	95
156	0.50	0.005	0.01	40	47	55	64	79	93	123
157	0.55	0.050	0.10	16	19	23	29	37	45	62
158	0.55	0.025	0.05	21	24	29	35	44	53	71
159	0.55	0.005	0.01	31	36	42	49	60	71	92
160	0.60	0.050	0.10	13	16	19	23	29	35	48
161	0.60	0.025	0.05	17	20	23	28	35	41	55
162	0.60	0.005	0.01	25	29	33	39	47	55	72
163	0.65	0.050	0.10	11	13	15	19	23	28	38
164	0.65	0.025	0.05	14	16	19	22	28	33	44
165	0.65	0.005	0.01	21	24	27	31	38	44	57
166	0.70	0.050	0.10	9	11	13	15	19	23	31
167	0.70	0.025	0.05	12	14	16	19	23	27	36
168	0.70	0.005	0.01	17	20	22	26	31	36	46

Table 10.4 (*continued*)

$P_1 = .25$

Row	P_2	α 1-Tail	α 2-Tail	POWER (%) 50	60	70	80	90	95	99
169	0.26	0.050	0.10	10431	13887	18091	23718	32728	41324	60140
170	0.25	0.025	0.05	14796	18807	23562	30051	40108	49576	70024
171	0.26	0.005	0.01	25295	30479	36595	44458	56545	67700	91309
172	0.27	0.050	0.10	2703	3565	4629	6054	8334	10510	15273
173	0.27	0.025	0.05	3795	4811	6040	7657	10203	12600	17775
174	0.27	0.005	0.01	6454	7766	9314	11305	14365	17188	23164
175	0.28	0.050	0.10	1238	1625	2104	2745	3771	4749	5891
176	0.28	0.025	0.05	1729	2186	2739	3466	4611	5689	8017
177	0.28	0.005	0.01	2926	3516	4212	5107	6484	7753	10441
178	0.29	0.050	0.10	716	937	1210	1574	2158	2714	3933
179	0.29	0.025	0.05	996	1256	1571	1985	2636	3249	4573
180	0.29	0.005	0.01	1677	2013	2409	2919	3702	4424	5953
181	0.30	0.050	0.10	471	614	790	1026	1404	1764	2552
182	0.30	0.025	0.05	653	821	1024	1292	1714	2110	2967
183	0.30	0.005	0.01	1094	1311	1567	1897	2403	2871	3860
184	0.35	0.050	0.10	133	171	217	279	378	472	678
185	0.35	0.025	0.05	181	225	279	349	459	563	787
186	0.35	0.005	0.01	298	355	422	508	641	763	1022
187	0.40	0.050	0.10	66	83	105	133	179	222	317
188	0.40	0.025	0.05	88	109	133	166	216	264	367
189	0.40	0.005	0.01	142	169	200	239	300	357	476
190	0.45	0.050	0.10	41	51	63	80	106	131	185
191	0.45	0.025	0.05	54	66	80	98	128	155	214
192	0.45	0.005	0.01	85	101	118	141	177	209	277
193	0.50	0.050	0.10	28	35	43	54	71	87	122
194	0.50	0.025	0.05	37	45	54	66	85	103	141
195	0.50	0.005	0.01	58	68	79	94	117	138	183
196	0.55	0.050	0.10	21	26	31	39	51	62	87
197	0.55	0.025	0.05	27	33	39	48	61	73	100
198	0.55	0.005	0.01	42	49	57	68	84	98	129
199	0.60	0.050	0.10	17	20	24	30	38	46	64
200	0.60	0.025	0.05	21	25	30	36	46	55	74
201	0.60	0.005	0.01	32	37	43	51	63	73	96
202	0.65	0.050	0.10	13	16	19	23	30	36	49
203	0.65	0.025	0.05	17	20	24	28	36	43	57
204	0.65	0.005	0.01	26	30	34	40	49	57	74
205	0.70	0.050	0.10	11	13	16	19	24	29	39
206	0.70	0.025	0.05	14	16	19	23	28	34	45
207	0.70	0.005	0.01	21	24	28	32	39	45	58
208	0.75	0.050	0.10	9	11	13	16	19	23	31
209	0.75	0.025	0.05	12	14	16	19	23	27	36
210	0.75	0.005	0.01	17	20	23	26	31	36	46

Table 10.4 (*continued*)

		α		POWER (%)						
				$P_1 = .3$						
Row	P_2	*1-Tail*	*2-Tail*	50	60	70	80	90	95	99
211	0.31	0.050	0.10	11672	15472	20163	26442	36495	46086	67081
212	0.31	0.025	0.05	16486	20962	26379	33508	44730	55294	78110
213	0.31	0.005	0.01	28202	33986	40810	49583	63071	75517	101860
214	0.32	0.050	0.10	2994	3952	5136	6719	9255	11674	15969
215	0.32	0.025	0.05	4208	5337	6704	8502	11332	13997	19751
216	0.32	0.005	0.01	7164	8623	10344	12557	15959	19098	25742
217	0.33	0.050	0.10	1364	1794	2324	3034	4170	5254	7627
218	0.33	0.025	0.05	1909	2415	3027	3833	5102	6296	8874
219	0.33	0.005	0.01	3234	3888	4659	5651	7176	8582	11560
220	0.34	0.050	0.10	786	1030	1330	1733	2377	2992	4337
221	0.34	0.025	0.05	1095	1382	1729	2186	2905	3582	5044
222	0.34	0.005	0.01	1847	2218	2655	3217	4082	4879	6567
223	0.35	0.050	0.10	515	672	866	1125	1541	1937	2805
224	0.35	0.025	0.05	714	899	1123	1418	1882	2318	3261
225	0.35	0.005	0.01	1199	1438	1721	2083	2641	3155	4243
226	0.40	0.050	0.10	143	184	234	301	408	510	734
227	0.40	0.025	0.05	195	243	300	377	496	609	852
228	0.40	0.005	0.01	321	382	455	549	693	825	1106
229	0.45	0.050	0.10	70	88	111	141	190	236	338
230	0.45	0.025	0.05	93	115	142	176	230	281	392
231	0.45	0.005	0.01	151	179	212	255	320	380	508
232	0.50	0.050	0.10	42	53	66	83	111	137	195
233	0.50	0.025	0.05	56	69	84	103	134	163	226
234	0.50	0.005	0.01	89	106	124	149	186	220	292
235	0.55	0.050	0.10	29	36	44	56	73	90	127
236	0.55	0.025	0.05	38	46	56	69	88	107	147
237	0.55	0.005	0.01	60	70	82	98	122	144	190
238	0.60	0.050	0.10	22	26	32	40	52	64	89
239	0.60	0.025	0.05	28	33	40	49	63	75	103
240	0.60	0.005	0.01	43	50	59	70	86	101	133
241	0.65	0.050	0.10	17	20	24	30	39	47	66
242	0.65	0.025	0.05	21	26	30	37	47	56	76
243	0.65	0.005	0.01	33	38	44	52	64	75	98
244	0.70	0.050	0.10	13	16	19	23	30	36	50
245	0.70	0.025	0.05	17	20	24	29	36	43	58
246	0.70	0.005	0.01	26	30	34	40	49	57	75
247	0.75	0.050	0.10	11	13	16	19	24	29	39
248	0.75	0.025	0.05	14	16	19	23	28	34	45
249	0.75	0.005	0.01	21	24	28	32	39	45	58
250	0.80	0.050	0.10	9	11	13	15	19	23	31
251	0.80	0.025	0.05	12	14	16	19	23	27	36
252	0.80	0.005	0.01	17	20	22	26	31	36	46

Table 10.4 (*continued*)

$P_1 = .35$

		α		POWER (%)						
Row	P_2	*1-Tail*	*2-Tail*	50	60	70	80	90	95	99
253	0.36	0.050	0.10	12592	16697	21764	28547	39406	49767	72446
254	0.36	0.025	0.05	17793	22627	28479	36179	48302	59713	84359
255	0.36	0.005	0.01	30447	36695	44067	53543	68113	81557	110014
256	0.37	0.050	0.10	3217	4250	5524	7230	9961	12567	18271
257	0.37	0.025	0.05	4525	5742	7213	9150	12199	15069	21267
258	0.37	0.005	0.01	7709	9281	11134	13518	17182	20564	27720
259	0.38	0.050	0.10	1460	1922	2491	3254	4475	5639	8188
260	0.38	0.025	0.05	2045	2589	3247	4112	5475	6758	9528
261	0.38	0.005	0.01	3469	4171	5000	6065	7703	9214	12413
262	0.39	0.050	0.10	838	1099	1422	1853	2543	3201	4643
263	0.39	0.025	0.05	1169	1477	1849	2338	3109	3834	5400
264	0.39	0.005	0.01	1975	2372	2841	3443	4369	5224	7032
265	0.40	0.050	0.10	547	715	922	1200	1644	2067	2994
266	0.40	0.025	0.05	760	958	1197	1512	2008	2474	3481
267	0.40	0.005	0.01	1279	1534	1836	2223	2819	3368	4531
268	0.45	0.050	0.10	150	193	246	316	429	537	773
269	0.45	0.025	0.05	204	255	316	396	522	641	898
270	0.45	0.005	0.01	337	402	479	578	730	870	1166
271	0.50	0.050	0.10	72	91	115	147	198	246	352
272	0.50	0.025	0.05	97	120	147	183	240	293	408
273	0.50	0.005	0.01	157	186	221	265	333	396	529
274	0.55	0.050	0.10	43	54	68	86	114	142	201
275	0.55	0.025	0.05	58	70	86	106	138	168	233
276	0.55	0.005	0.01	92	109	128	153	191	227	301
277	0.60	0.050	0.10	30	37	45	57	75	92	130
278	0.60	0.025	0.05	39	47	57	70	90	109	150
279	0.60	0.005	0.01	61	72	84	100	124	147	194
280	0.65	0.050	0.10	22	27	32	40	53	64	90
281	0.65	0.025	0.05	28	34	41	49	63	76	104
282	0.65	0.005	0.01	44	51	59	70	87	102	135
283	0.70	0.050	0.10	17	20	24	30	39	47	66
284	0.70	0.025	0.05	21	26	30	37	47	56	76
285	0.70	0.005	0.01	33	38	44	52	64	75	98
286	0.75	0.050	0.10	13	16	19	23	30	36	49
287	0.75	0.025	0.05	17	20	24	28	36	43	57
288	0.75	0.005	0.01	26	30	34	40	49	57	74
289	0.80	0.050	0.10	11	13	15	19	23	28	38
290	0.80	0.025	0.05	14	16	19	22	28	33	44
291	0.80	0.005	0.01	21	24	27	31	38	44	57
292	0.85	0.050	0.10	9	11	13	15	19	22	30
293	0.85	0.025	0.05	12	13	15	18	22	26	35
294	0.85	0.005	0.01	17	19	22	25	30	35	45

Table 10.4 (*continued*)

$P_1 = .4$

		α		POWER (%)						
Row	P_2	*1-Tail*	*2-Tail*	50	60	70	80	90	95	99
295	0.41	0.050	0.10	13241	17561	22894	30033	41460	52364	76232
296	0.41	0.025	0.05	18715	23803	29961	38065	50823	62832	88770
297	0.41	0.005	0.01	32033	38608	46366	56339	71672	85821	115769
298	0.42	0.050	0.10	3373	4457	5795	7586	10453	13189	19178
299	0.42	0.025	0.05	4746	6023	7568	9602	12803	15816	22324
300	0.42	0.005	0.01	8089	9739	11685	14188	18035	21585	29099
301	0.43	0.050	0.10	1526	2010	2607	3405	4684	5904	8574
302	0.43	0.025	0.05	2139	2709	3398	4304	5732	7075	9977
303	0.43	0.005	0.01	3630	4366	5234	6350	8065	9648	12999
304	0.44	0.050	0.10	874	1147	1483	1934	2655	3344	4850
305	0.44	0.025	0.05	1220	1541	1930	2441	3247	4005	5642
306	0.44	0.005	0.01	2061	2477	2966	3596	4564	5457	7347
307	0.45	0.050	0.10	569	744	960	1249	1712	2154	3120
308	0.45	0.025	0.05	791	997	1247	1575	2092	2578	3628
309	0.45	0.005	0.01	1331	1598	1912	2316	2937	3510	4723
310	0.50	0.050	0.10	154	198	253	326	442	553	797
311	0.50	0.025	0.05	210	262	325	408	538	661	925
312	0.50	0.005	0.01	347	414	494	595	752	896	1202
313	0.55	0.050	0.10	73	93	117	150	202	251	359
314	0.55	0.025	0.05	99	122	150	187	244	299	416
315	0.55	0.005	0.01	160	190	225	270	340	404	540
316	0.60	0.050	0.10	44	55	68	87	115	143	203
317	0.60	0.025	0.05	58	71	87	107	140	170	235
318	0.60	0.005	0.01	93	110	129	154	193	229	304
319	0.65	0.050	0.10	30	37	45	57	75	92	130
320	0.65	0.025	0.05	39	47	57	70	90	109	150
321	0.65	0.005	0.01	61	72	84	100	124	147	194
322	0.70	0.050	0.10	22	26	32	40	52	64	89
323	0.70	0.025	0.05	28	33	40	49	63	75	103
324	0.70	0.005	0.01	43	50	59	70	86	101	133
325	0.75	0.050	0.10	17	20	24	30	38	46	64
326	0.75	0.025	0.05	21	25	30	36	46	55	74
327	0.75	0.005	0.01	32	37	43	51	63	73	96
328	0.80	0.050	0.10	13	16	19	23	29	35	48
329	0.80	0.025	0.05	17	20	23	28	35	41	55
330	0.80	0.005	0.01	25	29	33	39	47	55	72
331	0.85	0.050	0.10	11	13	15	18	23	27	37
332	0.85	0.025	0.05	13	16	18	22	27	32	42
333	0.85	0.005	0.01	20	23	26	30	37	42	54
334	0.90	0.050	0.10	9	10	12	14	18	21	28
335	0.90	0.025	0.05	11	13	15	17	21	25	33
336	0.90	0.005	0.01	16	18	21	24	29	33	42

Table 10.4 (*continued*)

				$P_1 = .45$						
		α		POWER (%)						
Row	P_2	*1-Tail*	*2-Tail*	50	60	70	80	90	95	99
337	0.46	0.050	0.10	13620	18066	23553	30899	42659	53880	78441
338	0.46	0.025	0.05	19252	24488	30826	39165	52293	64651	91343
339	0.46	0.005	0.01	32957	39724	47707	57970	73748	88309	119127
340	0.47	0.050	0.10	3461	4574	5948	7787	10732	13541	19691
341	0.47	0.025	0.05	4871	6182	7769	9857	13144	16238	22921
342	0.47	0.005	0.01	8303	9998	11997	14566	18517	22163	29879
343	0.48	0.050	0.10	1562	2058	2569	3438	4798	6048	8784
344	0.48	0.025	0.05	2190	2774	3480	4409	5872	7249	10222
345	0.48	0.005	0.01	3718	4472	5362	6505	8263	9885	13319
346	0.49	0.050	0.10	892	1171	1516	1977	2714	3418	4958
347	0.49	0.025	0.05	1246	1575	1972	2495	3319	4094	5768
348	0.49	0.005	0.01	2107	2531	3032	3676	4666	5579	7512
349	0.50	0.050	0.10	580	758	979	1274	1746	2197	3183
350	0.50	0.025	0.05	806	1017	1271	1607	2134	2630	3702
351	0.50	0.005	0.01	1358	1630	1950	2363	2997	3581	4819
352	0.55	0.050	0.10	155	200	255	329	446	559	805
353	0.55	0.025	0.05	212	265	328	412	543	667	934
354	0.55	0.005	0.01	350	418	498	601	759	905	1214
355	0.60	0.050	0.10	73	93	117	150	202	251	359
356	0.60	0.025	0.05	99	122	150	187	244	299	416
357	0.60	0.005	0.01	160	190	225	270	340	404	540
358	0.65	0.050	0.10	43	54	68	86	114	142	201
359	0.65	0.025	0.05	58	70	86	106	138	168	233
360	0.65	0.005	0.01	92	109	128	153	191	227	301
361	0.70	0.050	0.10	29	36	44	56	73	90	127
362	0.70	0.025	0.05	38	46	56	69	88	107	147
363	0.70	0.005	0.01	60	70	82	98	122	144	190
364	0.75	0.050	0.10	21	26	31	39	51	62	87
365	0.75	0.025	0.05	27	33	39	48	61	73	100
366	0.75	0.005	0.01	42	49	57	68	84	98	129
367	0.80	0.050	0.10	16	19	23	29	37	45	62
368	0.80	0.025	0.05	21	24	29	35	44	53	71
369	0.80	0.005	0.01	31	36	42	49	60	71	92
370	0.85	0.050	0.10	13	15	18	22	28	33	46
371	0.85	0.025	0.05	16	19	22	26	33	39	53
372	0.85	0.005	0.01	24	28	32	37	45	52	68
373	0.90	0.050	0.10	10	12	14	17	21	25	34
374	0.90	0.025	0.05	13	15	17	20	25	30	40
375	0.90	0.005	0.01	19	22	25	28	34	40	51
376	0.95	0.050	0.10	9	10	11	13	17	20	26
377	0.95	0.025	0.05	11	12	14	16	20	23	30
378	0.95	0.005	0.01	15	17	20	22	27	31	39

Table 10.4 (continued)

$P_1 = .5$										
		α		POWER (%)						
Row	P_2	1-Tail	2-Tail	50	60	70	80	90	95	99
379	0.51	0.050	0.10	13729	18210	23742	31147	43001	54313	79072
380	0.51	0.025	0.05	19406	24684	31073	39479	52713	65171	92078
381	0.51	0.005	0.01	33221	40043	48090	58436	74341	89019	120086
382	0.52	0.050	0.10	3481	4601	5983	7834	10796	13622	19809
383	0.52	0.025	0.05	4900	6219	7815	9916	13223	16336	23059
384	0.52	0.005	0.01	8353	10058	12068	14654	18628	22296	30058
385	0.53	0.050	0.10	1568	2066	2680	3502	4817	6072	8819
386	0.53	0.025	0.05	2199	2785	3494	4427	5895	7278	10263
387	0.53	0.005	0.01	3733	4490	5383	6531	8296	9925	13372
388	0.54	0.050	0.10	894	1174	1519	1980	2720	3425	4968
389	0.54	0.025	0.05	1249	1578	1976	2500	3326	4102	5779
390	0.54	0.005	0.01	2111	2536	3038	3683	4675	5590	7527
391	0.55	0.050	0.10	580	758	979	1274	1746	2197	3183
392	0.55	0.025	0.05	806	1017	1271	1607	2134	2630	3702
393	0.55	0.005	0.01	1358	1630	1950	2363	2997	3581	4819
394	0.60	0.050	0.10	154	198	253	326	442	553	797
395	0.60	0.025	0.05	210	262	325	408	538	661	925
396	0.60	0.005	0.01	347	414	494	595	752	896	1202
397	0.65	0.050	0.10	72	91	115	147	198	246	352
398	0.65	0.025	0.05	97	120	147	183	240	293	408
399	0.65	0.005	0.01	157	186	221	265	333	396	529
400	0.70	0.050	0.10	42	53	66	83	111	137	195
401	0.70	0.025	0.05	56	69	84	103	134	163	226
402	0.70	0.005	0.01	89	106	124	149	186	220	292
403	0.75	0.050	0.10	28	35	43	54	71	87	122
404	0.75	0.025	0.05	37	45	54	66	85	103	141
405	0.75	0.005	0.01	58	68	79	94	117	138	183
406	0.80	0.050	0.10	20	25	30	37	48	59	82
407	0.80	0.025	0.05	26	31	37	45	58	70	95
408	0.80	0.005	0.01	40	47	55	64	79	93	123
409	0.85	0.050	0.10	15	18	22	27	35	42	58
410	0.85	0.025	0.05	20	23	27	33	42	50	67
411	0.85	0.005	0.01	30	34	39	46	57	66	86
412	0.90	0.050	0.10	12	14	17	20	26	31	42
413	0.90	0.025	0.05	15	18	21	25	31	36	49
414	0.90	0.005	0.01	23	26	30	34	42	48	62
415	0.95	0.050	0.10	10	11	13	16	20	23	31
416	0.95	0.025	0.05	12	14	16	19	23	27	36
417	0.95	0.005	0.01	18	20	23	26	31	36	46
418	1.00	0.050	0.10	8	9	11	12	15	18	23
419	1.00	0.025	0.05	10	11	13	15	18	21	27
420	1.00	0.005	0.01	14	16	18	20	24	27	34

Table 10.4 (*continued*)

$P_1 = .55$

		α		POWER (%)						
Row	P_2	*1-Tail*	*2-Tail*	50	60	70	80	90	95	99
421	0.56	0.050	0.10	13566	17994	23459	30775	42488	53663	78125
422	0.56	0.025	0.05	19176	24390	30702	39008	52083	64391	90975
423	0.56	0.005	0.01	32825	39564	47515	57737	73452	87953	118647
424	0.57	0.050	0.10	3434	4538	5901	7725	10646	13433	19533
425	0.57	0.025	0.05	4833	6133	7707	9779	13039	16108	22738
426	0.57	0.005	0.01	8237	9918	11901	14450	18369	21985	29639
427	0.58	0.050	0.10	1544	2034	2638	3447	4741	5976	8679
428	0.58	0.025	0.05	2165	2741	3439	4357	5802	7162	10100
429	0.58	0.005	0.01	3674	4419	5298	6428	8164	9767	13159
430	0.59	0.050	0.10	879	1153	1492	1946	2671	3364	4879
431	0.59	0.025	0.05	1227	1550	1941	2456	3266	4029	5676
432	0.59	0.005	0.01	2074	2491	2984	3618	4591	5490	7392
433	0.60	0.050	0.10	569	744	960	1249	1712	2154	3120
434	0.60	0.025	0.05	791	997	1247	1575	2092	2578	3628
435	0.60	0.005	0.01	1331	1598	1912	2316	2937	3510	4723
436	0.65	0.050	0.10	150	193	246	316	429	537	773
437	0.65	0.025	0.05	204	255	316	396	522	641	898
438	0.65	0.005	0.01	337	402	479	578	730	870	1166
439	0.70	0.050	0.10	70	88	111	141	190	236	338
440	0.70	0.025	0.05	93	115	142	176	230	281	392
441	0.70	0.005	0.01	151	179	212	255	320	380	508
442	0.75	0.050	0.10	41	51	63	80	106	131	185
443	0.75	0.025	0.05	54	66	80	98	128	155	214
444	0.75	0.005	0.01	85	101	118	141	177	209	277
445	0.80	0.050	0.10	27	33	41	51	66	82	114
446	0.80	0.025	0.05	35	42	51	62	80	97	132
447	0.80	0.005	0.01	55	64	75	89	110	130	171
448	0.85	0.050	0.10	19	23	28	35	45	55	76
449	0.85	0.025	0.05	25	29	35	42	54	65	88
450	0.85	0.005	0.01	38	44	51	60	74	86	113
451	0.90	0.050	0.10	14	17	21	25	32	38	53
452	0.90	0.025	0.05	18	21	25	30	38	45	61
453	0.90	0.005	0.01	27	32	36	42	52	60	78
454	0.95	0.050	0.10	11	13	16	19	23	28	38
455	0.95	0.025	0.05	14	16	19	22	28	33	43
456	0.95	0.005	0.01	21	24	27	31	38	43	56
457	1.00	0.050	0.10	9	10	12	14	17	21	27
458	1.00	0.025	0.05	11	13	15	17	21	24	31
459	1.00	0.005	0.01	16	18	20	23	28	32	40

Table 10.4 (*continued*)

$P_1 = .6$

Row	P_2	α 1-Tail	α 2-Tail	POWER (%) 50	60	70	80	90	95	99
460	0.61	0.050	0.10	13133	17417	22706	29785	41118	51931	75601
461	0.61	0.025	0.05	18561	23607	29714	37751	50402	62312	88035
462	0.61	0.005	0.01	31768	38289	45982	55873	71079	85111	114810
463	0.62	0.050	0.10	3319	4385	5701	7462	10282	12973	18862
464	0.62	0.025	0.05	4670	5925	7445	9445	12593	15556	21956
465	0.62	0.005	0.01	7957	9579	11494	13955	17738	21230	28620
466	0.63	0.050	0.10	1490	1962	2544	3323	4570	5760	8364
467	0.63	0.025	0.05	2088	2643	3315	4200	5592	6902	9732
468	0.63	0.005	0.01	3542	4260	5106	6195	7868	9412	12679
469	0.64	0.050	0.10	847	1111	1436	1872	2570	3235	4692
470	0.64	0.025	0.05	1181	1492	1868	2363	3142	3875	5458
471	0.64	0.005	0.01	1995	2397	2870	3479	4415	5279	7107
472	0.65	0.050	0.10	547	715	922	1200	1644	2067	2994
473	0.65	0.025	0.05	760	958	1197	1512	2008	2474	3481
474	0.65	0.005	0.01	1279	1534	1836	2223	2819	3368	4531
475	0.70	0.050	0.10	143	184	234	301	408	510	734
476	0.70	0.025	0.05	195	243	300	377	496	609	852
477	0.70	0.005	0.01	321	382	455	549	693	825	1106
478	0.75	0.050	0.10	66	83	105	133	179	222	317
479	0.75	0.025	0.05	88	109	133	166	216	264	367
480	0.75	0.005	0.01	142	169	200	239	300	357	476
481	0.80	0.050	0.10	38	48	59	74	98	121	171
482	0.80	0.025	0.05	50	61	74	92	118	144	198
483	0.80	0.005	0.01	80	94	110	131	164	193	256
484	0.85	0.050	0.10	25	31	38	47	61	75	104
485	0.85	0.025	0.05	33	39	47	57	73	88	121
486	0.85	0.005	0.01	50	59	69	81	100	118	156
487	0.90	0.050	0.10	18	21	26	32	41	49	68
488	0.90	0.025	0.05	23	27	32	38	49	58	79
489	0.90	0.005	0.01	34	40	46	54	66	78	101
490	0.95	0.050	0.10	13	16	19	22	28	34	46
491	0.95	0.025	0.05	17	19	23	27	34	40	53
492	0.95	0.005	0.01	25	28	32	38	46	53	69
493	1.00	0.050	0.10	10	12	14	16	20	24	32
494	1.00	0.025	0.05	13	15	17	20	24	28	37
495	1.00	0.005	0.01	18	21	24	27	32	37	47

Table 10.4 (*continued*)

$P_1 = .65$

		α		POWER (%)						
Row	P_2	*1-Tail*	*2-Tail*	50	60	70	80	90	95	99
496	0.66	0.050	0.10	12430	16481	21481	28175	38892	49117	71499
497	0.66	0.025	0.05	17562	22333	28108	35708	47671	58933	83256
498	0.66	0.005	0.01	30051	36217	43492	52845	67223	80491	108575
499	0.67	0.050	0.10	3136	4142	5383	7044	9704	12242	17797
500	0.67	0.025	0.05	4410	5595	7028	8914	11884	14679	20716
501	0.67	0.005	0.01	7511	9041	10847	13169	16737	20031	27001
502	0.68	0.050	0.10	1406	1850	2397	3130	4303	5423	7873
503	0.68	0.025	0.05	1968	2491	3123	3955	5265	6498	9160
504	0.68	0.005	0.01	3337	4012	4808	5832	7406	8859	11933
505	0.69	0.050	0.10	798	1045	1351	1760	2415	3039	4406
506	0.69	0.025	0.05	1112	1403	1756	2220	2951	3639	5125
507	0.69	0.005	0.01	1876	2252	2697	3268	4147	4957	6672
508	0.70	0.050	0.10	515	672	866	1125	1541	1937	2805
509	0.70	0.025	0.05	714	899	1123	1418	1882	2318	3261
510	0.70	0.005	0.01	1199	1438	1721	2083	2641	3155	4243
511	0.75	0.050	0.10	133	171	217	279	378	472	678
512	0.75	0.025	0.05	181	225	279	349	459	563	787
513	0.75	0.005	0.01	298	355	422	508	641	763	1022
514	0.80	0.050	0.10	61	77	96	122	163	203	289
515	0.80	0.025	0.05	81	100	122	152	198	241	334
516	0.80	0.005	0.01	131	154	183	219	274	325	433
517	0.85	0.050	0.10	35	43	54	67	89	109	154
518	0.85	0.025	0.05	46	56	67	83	107	129	178
519	0.85	0.005	0.01	72	85	99	118	147	173	229
520	0.90	0.050	0.10	23	28	34	42	54	66	92
521	0.90	0.025	0.05	29	35	42	51	65	78	106
522	0.90	0.005	0.01	45	52	61	72	89	104	136
523	0.95	0.050	0.10	16	19	23	28	35	43	58
524	0.95	0.025	0.05	20	24	28	34	42	50	67
525	0.95	0.005	0.01	30	35	40	47	57	67	86
526	1.00	0.050	0.10	12	14	16	19	24	29	38
527	1.00	0.025	0.05	15	17	20	23	29	34	44
528	1.00	0.005	0.01	21	24	28	32	38	44	57

Table 10.4 (continued)

$P_1 = .7$

		α		POWER (%)						
Row	P_2	1-Tail	2-Tail	50	60	70	80	90	95	99
529	0.71	0.050	0.10	11455	15184	19786	25947	35810	45220	65819
530	0.71	0.025	0.05	16179	20570	25885	32879	43890	54254	76640
531	0.71	0.005	0.01	27673	33348	40043	48651	61884	74096	99942
532	0.72	0.050	0.10	2885	3808	4947	6472	8912	11241	16338
533	0.72	0.025	0.05	4055	5142	6457	8188	10912	13477	19016
534	0.72	0.005	0.01	6900	8304	9961	12091	15366	18387	24783
535	0.73	0.050	0.10	1292	1698	2198	2869	3942	4966	7207
536	0.73	0.025	0.05	1806	2284	2862	3624	4821	5949	8384
537	0.73	0.005	0.01	3058	3675	4404	5340	6780	8109	10921
538	0.74	0.050	0.10	732	957	1236	1609	2206	2775	4021
539	0.74	0.025	0.05	1018	1284	1506	2029	2695	3322	4577
540	0.74	0.005	0.01	1715	2058	2463	2984	3785	4524	6088
541	0.75	0.050	0.10	471	614	790	1026	1404	1764	2552
542	0.75	0.025	0.05	653	821	1024	1292	1714	2110	2967
543	0.75	0.005	0.01	1094	1311	1567	1897	2403	2871	3860
544	0.80	0.050	0.10	121	155	196	251	339	423	607
545	0.80	0.025	0.05	164	203	251	314	412	505	705
546	0.80	0.005	0.01	268	319	379	456	574	683	914
547	0.85	0.050	0.10	55	69	86	108	144	179	254
548	0.85	0.025	0.05	73	89	108	134	174	212	294
549	0.85	0.005	0.01	116	137	161	193	241	286	380
550	0.90	0.050	0.10	31	38	47	59	77	94	132
551	0.90	0.025	0.05	41	49	59	72	92	111	152
552	0.90	0.005	0.01	63	74	86	102	126	149	196
553	0.95	0.050	0.10	20	24	29	36	46	55	77
554	0.95	0.025	0.05	26	30	36	43	55	65	88
555	0.95	0.005	0.01	39	45	52	61	74	87	113
556	1.00	0.050	0.10	14	16	19	23	29	35	47
557	1.00	0.025	0.05	17	20	24	28	34	41	54
558	1.00	0.005	0.01	25	29	33	38	46	54	69

$P_1 = .75$

		α		POWER (%)						
Row	P_2	1-Tail	2-Tail	50	60	70	80	90	95	99
559	0.76	0.050	0.10	10210	13527	17620	23099	31871	40241	58562
560	0.76	0.025	0.05	14412	18317	23045	29265	39058	48276	68186
561	0.76	0.005	0.01	24635	29682	35637	43293	55062	65923	88911
562	0.77	0.050	0.10	2567	3385	4394	5744	7906	9969	14484
563	0.77	0.025	0.05	3603	4566	5731	7264	9678	11950	16856
564	0.77	0.005	0.01	6124	7368	8835	10722	13623	16300	21965
565	0.78	0.050	0.10	1147	1505	1947	2539	3485	4388	6365
566	0.78	0.025	0.05	1601	2023	2533	3204	4261	5256	7404
567	0.78	0.005	0.01	2705	3250	3893	4719	5989	7161	9642
568	0.79	0.050	0.10	649	847	1092	1419	1944	2444	3538
569	0.79	0.025	0.05	900	1134	1416	1788	2374	2924	4114
570	0.79	0.005	0.01	1512	1814	2170	2628	3331	3980	5353
571	0.80	0.050	0.10	417	542	696	903	1233	1547	2237
572	0.80	0.025	0.05	576	723	901	1135	1503	1850	2599
573	0.80	0.005	0.01	961	1152	1376	1664	2107	2515	3380
574	0.85	0.050	0.10	106	135	170	217	292	364	521
575	0.85	0.025	0.05	143	176	217	270	354	433	603
576	0.85	0.005	0.01	231	275	326	392	492	585	782
577	0.90	0.050	0.10	48	59	73	92	121	150	211
578	0.90	0.025	0.05	62	76	92	113	146	177	244
579	0.90	0.005	0.01	98	115	136	162	201	238	316
580	0.95	0.050	0.10	27	32	39	48	63	76	106
581	0.95	0.025	0.05	34	41	49	59	75	90	122
582	0.95	0.005	0.01	52	61	70	83	102	120	157
583	1.00	0.050	0.10	17	20	24	29	36	43	59
584	1.00	0.025	0.05	21	25	29	34	43	51	68
585	1.00	0.005	0.01	31	36	41	47	58	67	86

Table 10.4 (*continued*)

$P_1 = .8$

Row	P_2	α 1-Tail	α 2-Tail	POWER (%) 50	60	70	80	90	95	99
586	0.81	0.050	0.10	8695	11509	14983	19633	27077	34180	49727
587	0.81	0.025	0.05	12260	15575	19586	24865	33176	40998	57894
588	0.81	0.005	0.01	20936	25219	30273	36769	46757	55974	75482
589	0.82	0.050	0.10	2182	2871	3723	4862	6686	8427	12236
590	0.82	0.025	0.05	3056	3868	4851	6145	8181	10098	14237
591	0.82	0.005	0.01	5182	6232	7470	9062	11510	13768	18548
592	0.83	0.050	0.10	973	1273	1644	2140	2933	3691	5348
593	0.83	0.025	0.05	1353	1707	2135	2698	3584	4418	6220
594	0.83	0.005	0.01	2280	2737	3276	3968	5033	6016	8096
595	0.84	0.050	0.10	549	714	918	1191	1628	2045	2956
596	0.84	0.025	0.05	758	953	1189	1498	1986	2445	3436
597	0.84	0.005	0.01	1269	1520	1817	2198	2784	3325	4469
598	0.85	0.050	0.10	352	455	583	754	1027	1288	1858
599	0.85	0.025	0.05	483	605	753	946	1251	1538	2158
600	0.85	0.005	0.01	803	960	1146	1384	1751	2089	2804
601	0.90	0.050	0.10	88	111	139	177	237	293	418
602	0.90	0.025	0.05	118	144	177	219	286	349	484
603	0.90	0.005	0.01	188	223	264	316	396	470	626
604	0.95	0.050	0.10	39	48	58	72	95	116	162
605	0.95	0.025	0.05	50	60	73	89	113	137	187
606	0.95	0.005	0.01	77	90	106	125	155	183	241
607	1.00	0.050	0.10	21	25	30	37	47	56	76
608	1.00	0.025	0.05	27	31	37	44	55	66	88
609	1.00	0.005	0.01	40	45	52	61	74	87	112

$P_1 = .85$

Row	P_2	α 1-Tail	α 2-Tail	POWER (%) 50	60	70	80	90	95	99
610	0.86	0.050	0.10	6909	9131	11875	15547	21426	27036	39314
611	0.86	0.025	0.05	9725	12342	15511	19680	26243	32421	45764
612	0.86	0.005	0.01	16577	19960	23950	29081	36969	44248	59655
613	0.87	0.050	0.10	1728	2268	2934	3825	5252	6614	9593
614	0.87	0.025	0.05	2412	3048	3817	4829	6421	7921	11159
615	0.87	0.005	0.01	4076	4897	5866	7111	9026	10792	14531
616	0.88	0.050	0.10	768	1001	1288	1672	2287	2873	4156
617	0.88	0.025	0.05	1063	1337	1668	2104	2791	3436	4831
618	0.88	0.005	0.01	1781	2134	2552	3088	3913	4674	6284
619	0.89	0.050	0.10	432	558	715	924	1259	1578	2276
620	0.89	0.025	0.05	593	742	922	1150	1533	1885	2644
621	0.89	0.005	0.01	984	1176	1403	1696	2144	2558	3435
622	0.90	0.050	0.10	276	354	451	580	787	984	1416
623	0.90	0.025	0.05	376	468	579	726	957	1174	1643
624	0.90	0.005	0.01	618	737	877	1058	1335	1591	2133
625	0.95	0.050	0.10	68	84	104	130	172	212	300
626	0.95	0.025	0.05	89	107	130	160	207	251	346
627	0.95	0.005	0.01	139	163	192	228	285	337	446
628	1.00	0.050	0.10	29	34	41	50	64	77	106
629	1.00	0.025	0.05	36	43	50	60	76	90	122
630	1.00	0.005	0.01	54	62	71	84	102	120	156

Table 10.4 (continued)

$P_1 = .9$

		α		POWER (%)						
Row	P_2	*1-Tail*	*2-Tail*	50	60	70	80	90	95	99
631	0.91	0.050	0.10	4851	6393	8296	10842	14919	18809	27324
632	0.91	0.025	0.05	6805	8620	10817	13708	18260	22544	31797
633	0.91	0.005	0.01	11557	13903	16670	20228	25698	30746	41429
634	0.92	0.050	0.10	1207	1574	2027	2633	3604	4530	6556
635	0.92	0.025	0.05	1672	2105	2628	3316	4399	5419	7621
636	0.92	0.005	0.01	2804	3363	4022	4869	6171	7372	9915
637	0.93	0.050	0.10	533	688	879	1135	1544	1935	2789
638	0.93	0.025	0.05	730	912	1133	1423	1880	2310	3238
639	0.93	0.005	0.01	1208	1443	1721	2078	2627	3134	4206
640	0.94	0.050	0.10	297	380	482	618	836	1043	1497
641	0.94	0.025	0.05	402	500	617	771	1014	1243	1736
642	0.94	0.005	0.01	657	783	930	1120	1412	1681	2251
643	0.95	0.050	0.10	189	239	300	382	513	638	911
644	0.95	0.025	0.05	252	311	382	475	621	758	1055
645	0.95	0.005	0.01	406	482	571	685	861	1023	1365
646	1.00	0.050	0.10	44	53	63	77	99	120	165
647	1.00	0.025	0.05	55	65	77	93	117	140	190
648	1.00	0.005	0.01	82	95	110	129	158	185	242

$P_1 = .95$

		α		POWER (%)						
Row	P_2	*1-Tail*	*2-Tail*	50	60	70	80	90	95	99
649	0.96	0.050	0.10	2522	3293	4245	5518	7556	9500	13755
650	0.96	0.025	0.05	3499	4407	5506	6951	9226	11367	15991
651	0.96	0.005	0.01	5876	7048	8432	10210	12944	15466	20806
652	0.97	0.050	0.10	616	789	1002	1286	1741	2175	3124
653	0.97	0.025	0.05	835	1038	1284	1606	2114	2592	3623
654	0.97	0.005	0.01	1367	1629	1938	2335	2945	3507	4699
655	0.98	0.050	0.10	266	334	417	529	706	876	1246
656	0.98	0.025	0.05	352	432	528	654	852	1039	1441
657	0.98	0.005	0.01	561	663	784	939	1177	1396	1861
658	0.99	0.050	0.10	145	178	218	272	358	440	619
659	0.99	0.025	0.05	187	226	272	333	429	519	713
660	0.99	0.005	0.01	289	338	397	471	586	692	916
661	1.00	0.050	0.10	89	107	129	158	204	247	342
662	1.00	0.025	0.05	112	133	158	190	242	290	393
663	1.00	0.005	0.01	167	193	225	265	326	382	502

For another example, return to Project 10.2, where we wished to estimate the difference between urban and rural children in the percentage having breathing problems. Suppose we wish to test to determine whether the defined parameters, denoted P_U and P_R, differed. We feel that urban children are more likely than rural children to have breathing problems, and we hope to show that our feeling is true. Thus, the hypotheses would be stated as $H_0: P_U = P_R$ and $H_a: P_U > P_R$. We decide that an important difference in the two rates is 5%: that is, if P_R exceeds P_U by at least 5%. We also choose $\alpha = .05$ and $\beta = .10$. We guess that $P_U = .15$ and $P_R = .20$. Then, from Table 10.4, we see that $n = 1027$, meaning that about 1027 rural and urban children would have to be studied to show a 5% difference between P_U and P_R. Note that in this one-tail test we could not possibly determine if $P_R > P_U$.

10.9 A NOTE ON SAMPLE SIZE TABLE FOR TESTING $H_0: P_1 - P_2$

A comparison of Table 10.4 with similar tables in other sources shows differences in the values of n. Recent research has improved the accuracy of estimates of n. The values of n in Table 10.4 reflect computations provided in references 1 and 2 and represent an adjustment to an earlier table of sample sizes in reference 3.

10.10 TESTING A HYPOTHESIS ABOUT $\mu_1 - \mu_2$

As in the earlier section on estimation, we shall consider the two designs: 1) one in which each experimental unit receives one factor level, and 2) a repeated measure design in which each experimental unit has the response variable measured under each factor level. Let us first consider the repeated measure design.

10.10.1 Repeated Measure Design

In Project 10.4, we estimated the difference (denoted $\mu_A - \mu_S$) in average FEV_1 between people breathing normal room air and people breathing air containing SO_2. Now we would like to determine whether μ_A and μ_S differ. The hypotheses to test are $H_0: \mu_A = \mu_S$ and the two-tail alternative $H_a: \mu_A \neq \mu_S$. As we did earlier, we must compute σ_D, and for that project, we estimated $\sigma_D = 1.5$. We also must determine how large a difference in liters between μ_A and μ_S is important. For this project, we decide that a .75 ℓ difference is important. If we call this difference the bound, B, we can again compute DELTA as B/σ or, for this example, DELTA $= .75/1.50 = .5$. We also choose $\alpha = .05$ and $\beta = .05$. We then can find the needed sample size in Table 10.5, where $n = 52$. Thus, about 52 people would be needed for detection of an average difference between μ_A and μ_S of .75 ℓ.

Let us return to Project 10.5 and try to determine whether the average IOP drops in glaucomatous beagles after they receive Drug A. If μ_N and μ_A represent the average IOP in beagles after they receive no drug and drug, respectively, we wish to test $H_0: \mu_N = \mu_A$ versus the one-tail alternative $H_a: \mu_N > \mu_A$, because we only are interested in showing that IOP is reduced after the drug is given. In that example, $\sigma_D = 2.5$. If we declare a .5 unit drop to be important, then DELTA $= .5/2.5 = .2$. If we choose $\alpha = .005$ and $\beta = .3$, we see from Table 10.5 that $n = 240$. We would have to study about 240 dogs to determine whether there was a .5 unit drop in IOP. This sample is very large, but we are trying to show a very small difference between the parameters, and α is chosen to be very small. To reduce the needed sample, we could increase the difference to be shown or α.

Table 10.5 Sample sizes required to test $H_0: \mu_1 = \mu_2$ for various α and power

		α		POWER (%)						
Row	*DELTA*	*1-Tail*	*2-Tail*	50	60	70	80	90	95	99
1	0.100	0.050	0.10	271	361	471	620	857	1083	1578
2	0.100	0.025	0.05	385	490	618	786	1051	1300	1838
3	0.100	0.005	0.01	661	797	958	1165	1484	1777	2399
4	0.125	0.050	0.10	174	231	302	397	548	693	1010
5	0.125	0.025	0.05	246	314	396	503	673	832	1177
6	0.125	0.005	0.01	423	511	614	746	950	1138	1535
7	0.150	0.050	0.10	121	161	210	276	381	482	702
8	0.150	0.025	0.05	171	218	275	350	467	578	817
9	0.150	0.005	0.01	294	355	426	518	660	790	1066
10	0.175	0.050	0.10	89	118	154	203	280	354	516
11	0.175	0.025	0.05	126	160	202	257	343	425	601
12	0.175	0.005	0.01	216	261	313	381	485	581	784
13	0.200	0.050	0.10	68	91	118	155	215	271	395
14	0.200	0.025	0.05	97	123	155	197	263	325	460
15	0.200	0.005	0.01	166	200	240	292	371	445	600
16	0.225	0.050	0.10	54	72	94	123	170	214	312
17	0.225	0.025	0.05	76	97	122	156	208	257	364
18	0.225	0.005	0.01	131	158	190	231	293	351	474
19	0.250	0.050	0.10	44	58	76	100	137	174	253
20	0.250	0.025	0.05	62	79	99	126	169	208	295
21	0.250	0.005	0.01	106	128	154	187	238	285	384
22	0.275	0.050	0.10	36	48	63	82	114	144	209
23	0.275	0.025	0.05	51	65	82	104	139	172	244
24	0.275	0.005	0.01	88	106	127	155	197	235	318
25	0.300	0.050	0.10	31	41	53	69	96	121	176
26	0.300	0.025	0.05	43	55	69	88	117	145	205
27	0.300	0.005	0.01	74	89	107	130	165	198	267
28	0.325	0.050	0.10	26	35	45	59	82	103	150
29	0.325	0.025	0.05	37	47	59	75	100	124	174
30	0.325	0.005	0.01	63	76	91	111	141	169	228
31	0.350	0.050	0.10	23	30	39	51	70	89	129
32	0.350	0.025	0.05	32	40	51	65	86	107	151
33	0.350	0.005	0.01	54	66	79	96	122	146	196
34	0.375	0.050	0.10	20	26	34	45	61	77	113
35	0.375	0.025	0.05	28	35	44	56	75	93	131
36	0.375	0.005	0.01	47	57	69	83	106	127	171
37	0.400	0.050	0.10	17	23	30	39	54	68	99
38	0.400	0.025	0.05	25	31	39	50	66	82	115
39	0.400	0.005	0.01	42	50	60	73	93	112	150
40	0.425	0.050	0.10	15	20	27	35	48	60	88
41	0.425	0.025	0.05	22	28	35	44	59	72	102
42	0.425	0.005	0.01	37	45	54	65	83	99	133
43	0.450	0.050	0.10	14	18	24	31	43	54	78
44	0.450	0.025	0.05	19	25	31	39	52	65	91
45	0.450	0.005	0.01	33	40	48	58	74	88	119
46	0.475	0.050	0.10	12	16	21	28	38	48	70
47	0.475	0.025	0.05	18	22	28	35	47	58	82
48	0.475	0.005	0.01	30	36	43	52	66	79	107
49	0.500	0.050	0.10	11	15	19	25	35	44	64
50	0.500	0.025	0.05	16	20	25	32	43	52	74
51	0.500	0.005	0.01	27	32	39	47	60	72	96
52	0.525	0.050	0.10	10	14	18	23	32	40	58
53	0.525	0.025	0.05	14	18	23	29	39	48	67
54	0.525	0.005	0.01	24	29	35	43	54	65	88
55	0.550	0.050	0.10	9	12	16	21	29	36	53
56	0.550	0.025	0.05	13	17	21	26	35	43	61
57	0.550	0.005	0.01	22	27	32	39	50	59	80
58	0.575	0.050	0.10	9	11	15	19	26	33	48
59	0.575	0.025	0.05	12	15	19	24	32	40	56
60	0.575	0.005	0.01	20	25	29	36	45	54	73
61	0.600	0.050	0.10	8	11	14	18	24	31	44
62	0.600	0.025	0.05	11	14	18	22	30	37	52
63	0.600	0.005	0.01	19	23	27	33	42	50	67
64	0.625	0.050	0.10	7	10	13	16	22	28	41
65	0.625	0.025	0.05	10	13	16	21	27	34	48
66	0.625	0.005	0.01	17	21	25	30	38	46	62
67	0.650	0.050	0.10	7	9	12	15	21	26	38
68	0.650	0.025	0.05	10	12	15	19	25	31	44

Table 10.5 (*continued*)

Row	DELTA	α 1-Tail	α 2-Tail	POWER (%) 50	60	70	80	90	95	99
69	0.650	0.005	0.01	16	19	23	28	36	43	57
70	0.675	0.050	0.10	6	8	11	14	19	24	35
71	0.675	0.025	0.05	9	11	14	18	24	29	41
72	0.675	0.005	0.01	15	18	22	26	33	39	53
73	0.700	0.050	0.10	6	8	10	13	18	23	33
74	0.700	0.025	0.05	8	10	13	17	22	27	38
75	0.700	0.005	0.01	14	17	20	24	31	37	49
76	0.725	0.050	0.10	6	7	9	12	17	21	31
77	0.725	0.025	0.05	8	10	12	15	20	25	35
78	0.725	0.005	0.01	13	16	19	23	29	34	46
79	0.750	0.050	0.10	5	7	9	12	16	20	29
80	0.750	0.025	0.05	7	9	11	14	19	24	33
81	0.750	0.005	0.01	12	15	18	21	27	32	43
82	0.775	0.050	0.10	5	6	8	11	15	19	27
83	0.775	0.025	0.05	7	9	11	14	18	22	31
84	0.775	0.005	0.01	11	14	16	20	25	30	40
85	0.800	0.050	0.10	5	6	8	10	14	17	25
86	0.800	0.025	0.05	7	8	10	13	17	21	29
87	0.800	0.005	0.01	11	13	15	19	24	28	38
88	0.825	0.050	0.10	4	5	7	10	13	16	24
89	0.825	0.025	0.05	6	8	10	12	16	20	28
90	0.825	0.005	0.01	10	12	15	18	22	27	36
91	0.850	0.050	0.10	4	5	7	9	12	15	22
92	0.850	0.025	0.05	6	7	9	11	15	18	26
93	0.850	0.005	0.01	10	12	14	17	21	25	34
94	0.875	0.050	0.10	4	5	7	9	12	15	21
95	0.875	0.025	0.05	6	7	9	11	14	17	25
96	0.875	0.005	0.01	9	11	13	16	20	24	32
97	0.900	0.050	0.10	4	5	6	8	11	14	20
98	0.900	0.025	0.05	5	7	8	10	13	17	23
99	0.900	0.005	0.01	9	10	12	15	19	22	30
100	0.925	0.050	0.10	4	5	6	8	11	13	19
101	0.925	0.025	0.05	5	6	8	10	13	16	22
102	0.925	0.005	0.01	8	10	12	14	18	21	29
103	0.950	0.050	0.10	3	4	6	7	10	12	18
104	0.950	0.025	0.05	5	5	7	9	12	15	21
105	0.950	0.005	0.01	8	9	11	13	17	20	27
106	0.975	0.050	0.10	3	4	5	7	10	12	17
107	0.975	0.025	0.05	5	6	7	9	12	14	20
108	0.975	0.005	0.01	7	9	11	13	16	19	26
109	1.000	0.050	0.10	3	4	5	7	9	11	16
110	1.000	0.025	0.05	4	5	7	8	11	13	19
111	1.000	0.005	0.01	7	8	10	12	15	18	24
112	1.025	0.050	0.10	3	4	5	6	9	11	16
113	1.025	0.025	0.05	4	5	6	8	10	13	18
114	1.025	0.005	0.01	7	8	10	12	15	17	23
115	1.050	0.050	0.10	3	4	5	6	8	10	15
116	1.050	0.025	0.05	4	5	6	8	10	12	17
117	1.050	0.005	0.01	6	8	9	11	14	17	22
118	1.075	0.050	0.10	3	4	5	6	8	10	14
119	1.075	0.025	0.05	4	5	6	7	10	12	16
120	1.075	0.005	0.01	6	7	9	11	13	16	21
121	1.100	0.050	0.10	3	3	4	6	8	9	14
122	1.100	0.025	0.05	4	5	6	7	9	11	16
123	1.100	0.005	0.01	6	7	8	10	13	15	20

10.10.2 No Repeated Measures

Extend Project 10.5 so that we now wish to estimate the average difference in IOP between the eyes of glaucomatous beagles receiving either Drug A or Drug B. Suppose that we now would like to determine whether there is a significant difference between μ_A and μ_B, the true mean IOP for Drug A and Drug B, respectively. The hypothesis to test is $H_0: \mu_A = \mu_B$ versus the two-tail alternative $H_a: \mu_A \neq \mu_B$. Each beagle was given only one drug: no repeated measures or blocking was employed. In that earlier example, we estimated $\sigma = 2.5$. We must decide how great a difference between μ_A and μ_B is important to detect; and for this example, we decide that a 2 unit difference is important. Then DELTA can be computed as DELTA $= B/\sigma = 2/2.5 = .8$. Finally, we must choose α and β. For this project, we choose $\alpha = .05$ and $\beta = .05$. Then, we can use Table 10.5 to determine n by finding the appropriate value and *doubling* it to indicate the number of beagles that must receive each drug. For DELTA $= .8$, $\alpha = .05$, and $\beta = .05$, we see from Table 10.5 that $n = 21$. Thus, $2n$ or 42 beagles would be needed in each drug group to answer the research hypothesis confidently.

As a final example, suppose that in Project 10.4 we wish to determine whether the average FEV_1 is higher for normals than for asthmatics while they are breathing air containing SO_2. Thus, if μ_N and μ_A represent the true average FEV_1 for normal and asthmatic people, respectively, we would like to test $H_0: \mu_N = \mu_A$ versus the one-tail alternative $H_a: \mu_N > \mu_A$. In that earlier example, we estimated $\sigma = 1$. We wish to detect a .5 difference if it exists, so DELTA $= .5/1 = .5$. For this one-tail test, we choose $\alpha = .05$ and $\beta = .2$. Thus, from Table 10.5, we see that $n = 25$ and $2n = 50$, so 50 normal and 50 asthmatic people would be needed to show the research hypothesis.

10.11 MORE THAN TWO FACTOR LEVELS

If you wish to compare more than two factor levels on either a nominal or a numerical response variable, the sample size estimation becomes much more difficult because the alternative hypothesis has many possibilities. You can obtain an approximation of the needed sample size by choosing two factor levels (the two most important, if a distinction can be made) and using our earlier discussion. This approximation will not be as accurate as earlier estimates, however, because adding additional factor levels influences the needed sample size. If possible, a professional statistician should be sought to provide advice on the needed sample size for this design. This same approach would be used if more than one factor were to be evaluated.

10.12 INTERESTING OBSERVATIONS ON SAMPLE SIZE ESTIMATION

In the various sample size estimations we have seen, the typical required sample size for a nominal response variable was much larger than that required for a numerical response variable. The reason is that a single nominal response variable measurement provides much less information than does a single numerical response variable measurement; hence, many more observations typically are needed to achieve the research objective if the response variable is on a nominal scale.

Second, the repeated measure design typically requires far fewer experimental units than does a similar design not using repeated measures. The reason is that each experimental unit in a repeated measure design is providing much additional information, and hence, fewer experimental units are required.

Note that in the sections where a repeated measure design was contrasted with a design using independent samples, the same tables were used for computing the sample size. However, for the independent samples design, the sample size in each group was twice that required for the repeated measure design, which meant a fourfold increase in the number of experimental units required for a study in which repeated measure was not employed. Thus, the repeated measure design can provide large budgetary savings in many studies.

10.13 SAMPLE SIZE IN STRATIFIED SAMPLING

In stratified sampling, you must determine how many experimental units to choose from each stratum. You must make three necessary considerations to arrive at the sample allocation: 1) the number or percentage of experimental units in each stratum, 2) the variability in the response variable in each stratum, and 3) the cost, in time and money, of measuring the response variable in each stratum. First, if one stratum has a great majority of the experimental units, then you should consider including a large proportion of those experimental units in the sample. This approach should provide a true cross section of the experimental units in the universe. Second, the variability in response variable measurements may differ among strata. If a particular stratum has more variability than do the other strata, you may wish to sample additional experimental units from that stratum. Finally, the cost of sampling among strata may vary. If the cost of sampling one particular stratum is higher than that of the others, you may decide to sample fewer experimental units from that stratum.

These considerations all affect the sample size determinations in stratified sampling. Be confident that you are choosing the *optimum* stratum sample sizes that will *maximize* the information you obtain. For more on this topic, see references 4 and 5.

10.14 SAMPLE SIZE IN CLUSTER SAMPLING

A researcher using cluster sampling has the responsibility of defining a cluster. Thus, you often will have to decide on the number of clusters that exist and the number of experimental units within each cluster. For example, if you wish to select a representative group of doctors in a particular state for interviews, cluster sampling would be beneficial if you must go to each doctor's office. You first would have to define the clusters in this study, which would be some breakdown into geographic regions. One possible definition of a cluster would be a county. If this unit were used as a cluster, a random sample of counties would be selected and then a random sample of doctors could be selected in each county. Another definition of a cluster could be a city, but this approach would exclude doctors not in cities from participating in the study. Thus, county would appear to be a logical definition of cluster unless you have a more appropriate geographic breakdown that includes all doctors.

A rule of thumb for defining the clusters is not to make the cluster sizes too large relative to the universe. If the cluster sizes are too large, the number of clusters will be small and the sampling of clusters may not result in a group representative of the entire universe. For more information on defining clusters, see references 4 and 5.

10.15 THE MAGICAL SAMPLE SIZE OF 30

Some researchers believe that, in any research project, a sample size of 30 for each factor level is sufficient. This idea probably is generated by an important theorem in statistics that is taught in many introductory statistics courses. The theorem shows that statistics computed from samples of at least 30 observations have some nice properties and, hence, samples of this size are desirable. Statistical procedures that are less restrictive in the assumptions required for the procedure to be valid often are available when sample sizes reach 30. *However*, all that this statement means is that a better statistical procedure may be available to us for the analysis. It does not provide any information as to whether or not this sample size is adequate to achieve the research objective.

There are occasions in laboratory experimentation on animals when a repeated measure design may require only 10 or 12 animals to achieve the research objective; and there are many instances, as you have seen, when many more than 30 observations are required to achieve the research objective.

Thus, you should remember that a sample of size 30 may prove beneficial in the choice of statistical analysis but provides no information as to the chances of achieving the research objective.

10.16 DETERMINING YOUR NEEDED SAMPLE SIZE

For your particular research project, consider the answer to the following questions and then find your needed sample size in the tables in this chapter.

- If the chosen response variable is discrete or continuous, how much variability is expected between individual response variable measurements? If this quantity is unknown, what is the range of measurements?
- What type of inference will be made: estimation or hypothesis testing?
- How great an effect is to be shown? (That is, how accurate an estimate, how large a difference between levels of a factor, etc.?)
- What is the confidence coefficient for my estimation inference? What are α and β for my hypothesis-testing inference?
- From a practical viewpoint, how large a sample can be taken?

10.17 KEY POINTS

Chapters 9 and 10 presented the information for determining the needed sample size for some simple research designs. You should determine this needed sample size before beginning the data collection, so that you are confident that enough information can be obtained to achieve the research objective. To determine the needed sample size for a research project, you must decide 1) whether the type of inference is estimation or hypothesis testing, 2) the amount of variability in a numerical response variable, 3) the size of the effect to be shown, and 4) suitable confidence coefficient or significance level and power. Remember that the sample size estimate should not be accepted as an absolute number, but instead as a ballpark figure.

REFERENCES

1. Fleiss, J. L. 1981. *Statistical methods for rates and proportions.* New York: Wiley.
2. Casagrande, J. T., Pike, M. C., and Smith, P. S. 1978. An improved approximate formula for calculating sample sizes for comparing two binomial distributions. *Biometrics* 34: 483–486.
3. Fleiss, J. L. 1973. *Statistical methods for rates and proportions.* New York: Wiley.
4. Levy, P. S., and Lemeshow, S. 1980. *Sampling for health professionals.* Belmont, Calif: Lifetime Learning Publications.
5. Mendenhall, W., Ott, L., and Scheaffer, R. L. 1971. *Elementary survey sampling.* North Scituate, Mass: Duxbury.

CHAPTER **11**

Step Seven: Assigning Treatments to Study Participants

11.1 INTRODUCTION

The design of the research project is now almost complete: the type of response variable to collect has been selected, the experimental units have been defined, their method of selection is outlined, and the number of experimental units needed has been considered. The factors for this project have been determined, and each factor has been identified as either observational or experimental. The difference between these types of factors is that the levels of observational factors already are assigned to the experimental units, while the researcher has the responsibility of assigning the levels of experimental factors to the experimental units. Examples of observational factors are sex, blood type, age, and location of tumor in cancer patients. Examples of experimental factors include type of drug for treating hypertension (A versus B), type of contraceptive used (which also could be an observational factor, depending on the design of the project), and length of time spent exercising in a therapy unit each day. For these and other experimental factors, it is the researcher's responsibility to assign the various factor levels to the experimental units.

The concept of randomization is very important in the design of a research project containing at least one experimental factor. The process of **choosing a representative sample of experimental units** and the process of **randomizing these experimental units to factor levels** are two distinct concepts in experimental design, and you must be able to distinguish between them. The purpose of choosing a representative sample of experimental units is to minimize the bias in the sample so that the conclusion determined by your sample data can be extrapolated to the entire population of numbers. The purpose of randomizing the experimental units into the various factor levels is to control for confounding of this experimental factor with other extraneous factors so that the comparison of the levels of the experimental factor will be valid. An example of confounding is as follows: Suppose we wish to compare two drugs (A and B) for their ability to reduce blood pressure. It is known that older adults have higher blood pressure than do young adults, and because we do not need to establish this fact, age would be considered an extraneous factor. Now, suppose a disproportionate number of older adults in the sample were assigned to Drug A, and hence, a disproportionate number of young adults receive Drug B. If the results of the study show that the people on Drug B have a significantly lower blood pressure, on the average, than do the people on Drug A, we do not know whether 1) Drug B is better than Drug A at reducing blood pressure or 2) the results are caused by the large number of young adults receiving Drug B. In this situation, the extraneous factor of age is said to be confounded with the factor of interest, which is the type of antihypertensive drug. The researcher must be careful in assigning treatments (factor levels) to experimental units to prevent the factor of interest from becoming confounded with an extraneous factor.

Confounding can be introduced into an experimental design in several ways. In this chapter, we shall identify these forms of confounding and determine how to avoid them. We shall look at the following situations separately, because each presents unique confounding problems: 1) there is one experimental factor, and each experimental unit receives one level of the factor; 2) there is one experimental factor, and each experimental unit receives more than one level of the factor; and 3) there is more than one experimental factor.

11.2 RANDOMIZATION IN THE PRESENCE OF A SINGLE EXPERIMENTAL FACTOR

If there is a single experimental factor to evaluate, a researcher can assign each experimental unit to receive either one or more levels of the factor. If each experimental unit receives only one factor level, the researcher should randomize the assignment of factor level while making sure that levels of extraneous factors are balanced over all levels of the factor of interest. If each experimental unit receives all factor levels, the order of assignment should be properly randomized so that any type of residual effect will be balanced over all factor levels. Finally, if more than one factor level is assigned to each experimental unit, but not all levels, the assignment scheme should insure that each factor level is observed equally often and each pair of factor levels occurs together equally often on experimental units in the study.

11.2.1 One Level Assigned to Each Experimental Unit

Let us begin this section with a simple example. We wish to compare two drugs, A and B, on 100 available patients in a local hospital. Each drug is designed to reduce a person's heart rate. We decide to assign 50 persons to receive each of the drugs. Here are a few ways of accomplishing this aim that would result in a randomization of patients to each of the drugs.

1. Place the patient's names in a hat. The first 50 names drawn will receive Drug A. The remaining 50 people will receive Drug B.
2. If the names are listed on a sheet of paper, start with the first name. Toss a coin and if the coin lands head up, assign Drug A to that person. If it lands tail up, assign Drug B. Repeat this coin tossing for each person until one group has 50 members. Then assign the remaining people to the other group. Note that this technique also would work well in an outpatient setting, where the researcher would include those people in the study who came into the clinic. As each one enters, a coin is tossed and the patient is placed into a study group determined by the result of the tossed coin.
3. If each patient has a hospital number or an identification number of some type, such as a social security number, that number could be used to randomize patients. If the last digit of the number is even, the patient is assigned to Drug A, whereas an odd last digit results in the patient receiving Drug B. This randomization procedure will be valid only if odd and even digits are equally likely to occur in the last position.
4. Procedure 2 has the disadvantage that it may combine the last five or 10 people into the same group. If these people come into the clinic together or are related, a potential bias may be created. Procedure 3 has the disadvantage that you may end up with unequal numbers in the two groups. One means of preventing these occurrences is to use the randomization technique proposed by Zelen in reference 14. This procedure involves first dividing the patients into 25 groups of four people. This division could be done sequentially (i.e., the first four people entering form group 1, the second four group 2, and so on). Then, within each group, patients are assigned to the factor levels so that there is an equal allocation for each factor level. You can do so by first looking at all possible orderings of Drug A and Drug B in groups of four. There are six possible orderings, as shown in Table 11.1.

   Next, randomly order the integers 1 through 6. Let us assume that this ordering is 4, 6, 2, 1, 5, 3. Then assign ordering 4 to group 1, ordering 6

Table 11.1 Orderings of drugs A and B in groups of four.

		ORDERING					
		1	2	3	4	5	6
PERSON IN GROUP	1	A	B	A	B	A	B
	2	A	B	B	A	B	A
	3	B	A	A	B	B	A
	4	B	A	B	A	A	B

to group 2, ordering 2 to group 3, ordering 1 to group 4, ordering 5 to group 5, and ordering 3 to group 6. The people in each group then are assigned to the appropriate drug. Then, again randomly order the integers 1 through 6 and assign those orderings to group 7 through 12. Repeat this process until all 25 groups have been assigned orderings.

Each of these randomization schemes is designed so that the resulting group of people receiving Drug A will be similar to the group of people receiving Drug B. One should note that randomizing patients does not guarantee that a similar grouping will occur. We may end up by chance with a majority of women in one group and men in the other, or older people in one group and younger people in the other. If we feel that the results of the study would not be valid in this situation, it will be necessary to randomize patients in such a way as to avoid confounding the experimental factor of drug type with extraneous factors such as sex and age.

11.2.2 Controlling for Extraneous Factors

Let us look at how to handle this situation by means of another example.

Project 11.1 Toothpaste comparison study

Refer to Project 3.4, which had as its objective **to compare a new toothpaste (Brand A) to an existing brand made by the same company (Brand B) and two competing commercial brands (Brand C and Brand D) for flavor acceptance and also gingivitis control.**

The group of people participating in this study will represent a volunteer sample, because people will be recruited through advertising in newspapers and by word of mouth. Thus, the participants may not be truly representative of the entire universe. Thus, we should try to determine potential biases in the sample, because they could affect the inferences that we shall make. For example, suppose we feel that a majority of the volunteers will be people who visit their dentists regularly, because these people care for their teeth and would be more interested in this study. Also, if the study occurs in a college town, more young people than older ones may tend to volunteer, because free toothpaste, toothbrushes, and dental examinations are being offered. In this case, if young people will react differently to the toothpastes from the way older people will, the results of the study will be biased. We need to identify and control for these potential biases, if possible.

Once the people are selected to participate in the study, we must assign each person to receive one of the four brands of toothpaste. Again, we are concerned with preventing the extraneous factors from becoming confounded with the experimental factor. For example, suppose a majority of people who visit their dentists regularly are assigned to Brand A and Brand B, while most of the people who do not visit their dentists regularly are assigned to Brand C and Brand D. The results might show Brands A and B superior to Brands C and D, but we would not know whether Brands A and B were really better or whether the effect resulted from the fact that people with a better attitude and healthier gums received Brands A and B. The purpose of randomizing people into groups is to prevent this kind of occurrence.

We could randomize patients into groups by placing four pieces of paper in a hat, one each labeled A, B, C, and D, and selecting a piece of paper for each person entering the study. The person receives the brand noted on the paper. The result should be four homogeneous groups balanced fairly well for the extraneous factors. However, a randomized assignment *does not guarantee* these results. It is possible that we might randomize young people or people who visit their dentist regularly into one or two brands. This problem can be avoided if the people to participate in the study have been identified before the study begins and their extraneous factor levels are known. Then, people are stratified into subgroups determined by the levels of the extraneous factors. For example, if age, sex, and visit to the dentist are extraneous factors, we first divide the people into six subgroups based on the two qualitative extraneous factors. The six subgroups would be

1. Males, visit dentist every six months
2. Males, visit dentist at least once a year
3. Males, visit dentist less than once a year
4. Females, visit dentist every six months
5. Females, visit dentist at least once a year
6. Females, visit dentist less than once a year

Then, within each of the six subgroups, we order people by age from youngest to oldest. The next step is to assign Brand A, B, C, or D randomly to the youngest person in subgroup 1. Then, we alternately assign brands A, B, C, D to succeeding people in each subgroup. We repeat the same process for the remaining subgroups, and the result will be a random assignment of people to brands controlled for the three extraneous factors. (See Table 11.2.)

In this manner, we are guaranteed that the four study groups will be homogeneous, at least for the extraneous factors that we have identified.

In general, when there are multiple extraneous factors, one first should divide them into qualitative and quantitative factors. Then the qualitative factors should be combined so they are treated as a single factor, with the new levels being all possible factor level combinations from the qualitative, extraneous factors. Then, within each level, order the experimental units according to the levels of the quantitative extraneous factors. If the levels of the experimental factor then are applied sequentially (A, B, C, A, B, C, and so on), the result will be that the experimental units are stratified across each of the extraneous factors.

Let us now look at another research design, one in which each experimental unit receives every level of the experimental factor, and evaluate the type of confounding that occurs with that design.

Table 11.2 Assignment scheme controlling for three extraneous factors

SUBGROUP																	
1			*2*			*3*			*4*			*5*			*6*		
Person	Age	Brand	Person	Age	Brand	Person	Age	Brand	Person	Age	Brand	Person	Age	Brand	Person	Age	Brand
C. B.	14	C	J. P.	16	A	P. M.	21	B	M. B.	18	C	D. D.	22	B	J. L.	19	D
R. K.	17	D	F. D.	17	B	H. W.	22	C	B. K.	19	D	J. B.	23	C	R. H.	23	A
M. B.	19	A	K. C.	21	C	T. G.	22	D	N. L.	22	A	C. C.	27	D	B. V.	24	B
C. C.	19	B	F. D.	22	D	H. W.	26	A	W. L.	23	B	W. G.	29	A	R. C.	24	C
B. S.	24	C	B. M.	27	A	B. V.	29	B	S. K.	28	C	Y. S.	36	B	M. C.	27	D
S. B.	31	D	D. S.	31	B	T. B.	30	C	H. D.	31	D	T. S.	38	C	R. G.	31	A
K. J.	32	A	D. W.	33	C	K. C.	30	D	H. M.	33	A	B. Y.	39	D	D. C.	32	B
M. H.	40	B	P. R.	34	D	S. C.	38	A	D. N.	34	B	W. J.	42	A	J. B.	36	C
N. N.	51	C	C. M.	37	A	R. B.	43	B	D. M.	35	C	D. K.	43	B	W. K.	40	D
C. K.	52	D	M. M.	42	B	R. M.	55	C	R. M.	37	D	S. S.	48	C	O. B.	41	A

11.2.3 Each Level Assigned to Every Experimental Unit

In the previous section, we used an example in which we wished to compare two drugs, Drug A and Drug B, on their ability to reduce heart rate, and each person was assigned to receive one drug. Suppose that we now decide to have each person receive both drugs, one at a time. This arrangement is an example of the repeated measure design (crossover) that was discussed in Chapter 7. In what order should each person receive the drugs? Should the order be the same for all people? The answer is that the order of assignment should be randomized for each person. One reason is to account for a possible residual effect of the drugs. If we decide to let the participants rest one week between drugs to let the effect of the first drug wear off, and if it takes two weeks for the drug to clear the body completely, then there will be a residual effect that will influence the heart rate after the second drug is given. Assume that Drug A is more effective than is Drug B at reducing heart rate and that Drug A always is given first. If the residual effect is present, the heart rate measurements under Drug B will be lower because of a residual effect rather than because Drug B is effective. However, the results will indicate that there is no difference between the two drugs. To avoid this confounding caused by a residual effect, we should randomize the order of the drugs for each person.

Toss a coin, and if it lands head up, assign Drug A first. Otherwise, assign Drug B first. This approach is an example of a **randomized block design.** A randomized block design is one in which an experimental unit (or groups of homogeneous experimental units) receive each level of the experimental factor in a randomly assigned order. (References 1, 2, and 3 deal with randomized block designs.)

Fatigue resulting from repetition of a response under multiple factor levels or education through the repetition also are common residual types of problems encountered. Note that the randomization scheme described here *does not* eliminate these possible confounding effects but merely attempts to balance them out over all the factor levels.

As we pointed out earlier, randomization does not guarantee that each drug will occur first an equal number of times. If only five people were included in our study of Drug A and Drug B, there is a 38% chance that one of these drugs will occur first either four or five times. If more than two drugs are included, one may occur first or second a disproportionate number of times. This occurrence would put that drug at a distinct advantage (or disadvantage). One possible assignment scheme (Table 11.3) would put Drug A and Drug B at a distinct advantage or disadvantage if there is any type of residual effect, because Drug A generally is given early and Drug B near the end.

This type of assignment is possible if the order of drugs is randomized. If we are concerned with a possible residual effect of some sort (that is, residual drug effect, fatigue, learning effect), we should use a **Latin square** design. The levels of the experimental factor still are randomized in a Latin square design, but with the constraint that each level of the factor must occur an equal number

Table 11.3 A randomized block layout

		PERSON				
		1	2	3	4	5
	1	A	E	D	A	C
	2	C	A	A	D	B
ORDER	3	E	D	B	E	A
	4	D	C	C	B	E
	5	B	B	E	C	D

of times at each order of administration. This method requires the number of experimental units to be an exact multiple of the number of levels of the experimental factor. One possible Latin square layout for Table 11.3 is given in Table 11.4.

Note that each person receives each factor level; but in addition, each factor level occurs at each order of administration. This method balances out any consistent residual effect over all factor levels. For more information on Latin square designs, see references 1 and 2, or almost any book on statistical design of experiments.

If some multiple of five people were participating in this study, each group of five people would form a 5 × 5 Latin square. This design is called a **changeover design.** (See reference 4.)

The Latin square and changeover designs still have a potential flaw if one or more levels of the factor has a residual effect on only the following measurement. For example, in Table 11.4, if only Drug A has a residual effect that will affect the next measurement, then the measurements on Drug C all will be affected because Drug C always follows Drug A except when Drug A occurs last. To avoid this problem, we need a design that is "balanced for first residuals": that is, one in which each level occurs after each other level an equal number of times.

Table 11.4 A Latin square layout

		PERSON				
		1	2	3	4	5
	1	A	B	D	E	C
	2	C	A	B	D	E
ORDER	3	E	C	A	B	D
	4	D	E	C	A	B
	5	B	D	E	C	A

Table 11.5 Assignment scheme balancing first residuals

		PERSON									
		1	2	3	4	5	6	7	8	9	10
ORDER	1	A	B	C	D	E	D	E	A	B	C
	2	B	C	D	E	A	C	D	E	A	B
	3	E	A	B	C	D	E	A	B	C	D
	4	C	D	E	A	B	B	C	D	E	A
	5	D	E	A	B	C	A	B	C	D	E

For the example outlined in Table 11.4, we would need 10 people (or a multiple of 10) to achieve balance for first residuals. One possible assignment scheme would be like that given in Table 11.5.

Note that Drug A is followed by every other drug twice. The same is true for all other drugs. Thus, if any drug does have a residual effect, that effect is not eliminated but is balanced over all remaining levels of the factor. The result is to minimize its effect on any one level. Designs also exist for balancing for second residuals as well. We shall not discuss these designs further, because they can get complicated and are not used frequently in practice. However, you may see references 4, 5, and 6 for more information on these topics.

Some projects involve more levels of a factor than can be assigned to a block or experimental unit. In this instance, one should consider incomplete block designs, insuring that each factor level is assigned equally often and each pair of factor levels occurs together in experimental units an equal number of times, if possible. References 2 and 4 cover such designs.

Let us now look at how to randomize experimental units to factor levels when more than one experimental factor is present.

11.3 RANDOMIZING IN THE PRESENCE OF MULTIPLE EXPERIMENTAL FACTORS

Suppose that in addition to comparing Drug A and Drug B on heart rate, we also wish to compare Diet X and Diet Y on heart rate in the same experiment. In this case, the experimental units must be randomized into two experimental factors. There are several ways to do so.

First, we could randomize people into a drug type and a diet type independently. The disadvantage of this procedure is that the number of people in the four subgroups may be very unequal. For example, we may wind up with a majority of people assigned to receive Drug A also assigned to receive Diet X. At the same time, the Drug B people would be receiving Diet Y. Thus, if we noted differences in the heart rates, we would not know whether these differences resulted from drug or diet.

A second method would be first to randomize people into the two drug types. Next, within each drug type, the people could be randomized into diet types. This approach would require randomizing each participant twice, as in the first method; but we could control the number of people receiving each diet and drug combination.

A third method of randomizing would be first to combine the two factors into a single factor:

Level 1:	Drug A, diet X
Level 2:	Drug A, diet Y
Level 3:	Drug B, diet X
Level 4:	Drug B, diet Y

Then, treating this combination as a single factor, randomize the patients into one of the four levels. This method requires only one randomization of the experimental units into the levels of the experimental factors. This technique will be more advantageous than the first two when there are three or more experimental factors. It also provides the researcher with more control over the number of people being assigned to each factor level.

It is an advantage in many research projects for the people serving as experimental units and the principal researcher not to know which levels of the experimental factors are assigned to whom. This concept is called *blinding* (or masking), and it will be discussed in the next section.

11.4. THE CONCEPT OF BLINDING

A series of experiments was conducted at the Hawthorne plant of the General Electric Company in the late 1920s. One conclusion from these studies was that the productivity of the workers involved in the studies increased, regardless of any stimulus that was provided. Thus, the **Hawthorne effect** was defined as the phenomenon whereby an experimental unit has his response variable influenced merely by being included in a study, even if no positive stimulus or treatment is given. Reference 7 describes the original study from which the Hawthorne effect has evolved. References 8 and 9 discuss this research in detail, while summaries of the research are provided in references 10 and 11.

You must measure this effect in a study so that the effect of a positive stimulus can be evaluated fairly. This Hawthorne effect can be measured through the use of a **placebo**, which is a treatment appearing similar to the real treatment of interest but having no medicinal qualities. For example, if we developed a new drug to relieve tension headaches, we would compare the results of a treatment group receiving the new treatment to those of a control group receiving a sugar pill that appeared similar to the new drug. The control group would allow us to measure the amount of relief obtained by people who merely were told they are being treated for tension headaches. Then we hope we could show that the treatment group did much better in obtaining headache relief. In a study like this, where existing treatments already may be available, we also would be interested in showing that the new drug is superior to alternatives.

Another example of the Hawthorne effect was illustrated in Project 4.3 in Chapter 4, where the objective was to evaluate an educational procedure for its influence on the prejudice of school children toward the physically handicapped. A control group was used in that study to measure the effect of the researcher's presence in the classroom on the children not receiving the new educational procedure.

In some studies, the researcher, as well as the participants, should be kept blinded to who is receiving which treatment. This **double blind** design should be used in studies where the researcher can have some effect on the response variable measurement. For example, in the toothpaste clinical trial experiment outlined in Project 3.4, gingivitis is a somewhat subjective measurement determined by the researcher. If we hope to show Brand A to be a superior toothpaste in fighting gingivitis, we might subconsciously choose the lower gingivitis score for a person using Brand A when his or her gingiva scale is in between two levels on the scale. On the other hand, we might subconsciously give a person receiving another brand of toothpaste the higher gingiva level. Thus, Brand A would have an unfair advantage over the other brands, and its chances of ending up as the best toothpaste would be enhanced.

Even if we have no control over the response variable measurements, we may tend to subconsciously give more attention or encouragement to those people who are receiving the preferred treatment. Again, in this situation, the treatment we preferred would have an unfair advantage over the other treatments.

To employ double blinding in a research project, we must see that the treatments all appear physically alike. This rule poses no problem if the treatment is a pill or some other form of medication. However, if the treatment is a type of surgery or a type of drug administration (such as intravenous or oral), we cannot be blinded to who is receiving which treatment. If we cannot be blinded to the treatment given and cannot remain totally uninvolved with the participants in the study, then at least we should make an effort to treat each participant similarly and to try to develop a response variable that is as objective as possible. One possibility would be to have someone else who is unfamiliar with the objective of the research project collect the response variable measurements.

One very important topic remains in the area of randomization of people to treatment groups. That topic is the ethical consideration of randomization in the event that some treatments clearly are not as good as the others, such as when a control group (or placebo) is used. The next section of this chapter will provide some insight into this topic.

11.5 ETHICAL CONSIDERATIONS OF RANDOMIZATION

In Chapter 1, we briefly described a project in which a researcher wished to evaluate the effectiveness of a nitroglycerin paste on patients in coronary critical care units. He wanted to compare it to the currently used nitroglycerin pill for survival rate of patients. He felt confident that his paste was superior to the pill currently in use, yet the final results showed more and earlier deaths among patients receiving the paste than among the ones on the currently used pill.

The reason for these results was that the patients were not randomized into the two treatment groups. As patients entered the hospital, the researcher placed them into one of the two treatment groups based on the severity of their illness. Because he was confident that his paste was the better of the two treatments, he made the correct moral decision to place the most critically ill patients on his paste and the less seriously ill patients on the current pill. However, this step invalidated any statistical comparison of the treatments, because treatment group now was confounded with level of critical illness.

This type of project poses a very interesting dilemma: Should one provide the best possible medical care without concern for proving that it is the best? Or should one allow some people to receive possibly less than the best medical care in the hopes of establishing scientifically that one form of care is better than another? There is a great deal of interest in this topic, and many arguments are made on both sides. We cannot get involved in this philosophical discussion in this text, but you must be aware that such a problem does exist. References 12 through 18 delve into this question more deeply. They include discussions both for and against randomization techniques.

If a control group is to receive a placebo in an experimental study, the participants must be advised that one of the treatments may not provide any benefit. The participants should not know which treatment is the placebo or whether or not they are receiving it, but they must be told that one of the treatments may be ineffective. The participants are advised of this fact in a letter of consent, which they must sign before being included in an experimental study.

11.6 OBTAINING APPROVAL TO USE HUMAN SUBJECTS

In any research project that involves humans as subjects of experimentation and where there is some risk to the participating subjects, you must obtain approval for the project from a local Institutional Review Board (IRB). The interpretation of a subject at risk by the Secretary of Health, Education, and Welfare in 1976 was

> ". . . any individual who may be exposed to the possibility of injury, including physical, psychological, or social injury, as a consequence of participation as a subject in any research, development, or related activity which departs from the application of those established and accepted methods necessary to meet his needs, or which increases the ordinary risks of daily life, including the recognized risks inherent in a chosen occupation or field of service."

The committee will review the protocol for the project and the degree of risk to which the experimental subject may be exposed. Specific information that must be furnished to the committee includes:

1. The number of experimental and control subjects to be involved, and a statement as to how they will be obtained. Indicate amount of monetary compensation, if any.
2. Identification of the agents and procedures to be used on human subjects
3. A statement of what is expected to be the potential benefit to the subject and to medical knowledge

INFORMED CONSENT FORM

The principal investigator must prepare in layman's language a narrative description of the planned procedure or treatment. This description should include the following elements of information:

1. A fair explanation of the procedures to be followed and their purposes, including identification of any procedures that are experimental
2. A description of any attendant discomforts and risks reasonably to be expected
3. A description of any benefits reasonably to be expected
4. A disclosure of any appropriate alternative procedures that might be advantageous for the subject
5. An offer to answer any inquiries concerning the procedures
6. An instruction that the person is free to withdraw his consent and to discontinue participation in the project or activity at any time without prejudice to the subject
7. A concluding sentence that reads, "I have read and understand the above described (medical) procedure in which I am to participate and have received a copy of this description."

This consent form must be submitted as part of the protocol to the IRB.

A copy of the above description, signed by the subject and witnessed, is to be placed in the respective hospital chart or experimental record of each subject, and a duplicate copy is to be retained by the patient.

4. A considered evaluation of the risks involved, documented, if necessary and possible, by literature references, together with a statement of precautions that will be taken to minimize these risks
5. A statement that informed consent will be obtained in accordance with governmental and local regulations for the protection of human subjects

Other information also may be requested, and you must realize that the proposed experimental study cannot begin until approval is obtained from this committee.

Specific guidelines to follow in developing the informed consent form are outlined in the accompanying approval form.

11.7 CHOOSING YOUR RANDOMIZATION TECHNIQUE

If there are any experimental factors in your research project, consider the following questions in determining how to randomize factor levels to experimental units.

- What are the experimental factors in this research project?
- What are the potential extraneous factors for which I must control?
- Will a repeated measure or blocking design be employed? (That is, will the individual experimental units or groups of homogeneous experimental units receive more than one factor level combination?)
- What randomization technique shall I use to assign the levels of the experimental factors to the experimental units?
- Should blinding of either the experimental units or the researcher be employed?
- Are there any moral or ethical considerations that should be weighed against the chosen randomization technique?
- Is it necessary to obtain approval for the use of human subjects? If so, has the approval been given?

11.8 KEY POINTS

This chapter discussed various randomization techniques for assigning levels of experimental factors to the experimental units. These randomization techniques are necessary to prevent confounding of the important experimental factors with other factors. In some experimental situations, however, the moral and ethical considerations require a hard look at whether randomization is feasible.

The concept of blinding also was discussed. In blinding, either the experimental unit (if a person) or the researcher does not know which level of the experimental factor is being assigned. This precaution prevents the experimental unit or researcher from unduly affecting the response variable measurement.

Finally, it was pointed out that the researcher must obtain approval to use human subjects in experimental studies. The information required to obtain this approval was outlined.

This chapter concludes the design stage of the research project. You should review all the important design considerations made thus far to be sure that all your decisions will result in a well-designed, efficient research project that will achieve the experimental objective. To facilitate this review, we list the considerations discussed in this text in Appendix A.

After you are satisfied with the design of the research project, the data collection could begin. However, it would be beneficial at this time to consider the statistical analysis that will achieve the research objective. Time can be saved and errors reduced if you think through this aspect of the project before the data collection begins.

For a discussion of the most commonly used statistical procedures to analyze biomedical research data, see reference 19. The discussion of each procedure centers on how to choose the appropriate analysis and how to interpret the results. You should determine whether one of these analyses is appropriate for your data. If a more complex analysis is needed, is it available with your computer software? Is someone competent in the use of the needed analysis available to perform and interpret it? Answers to the questions should be obtained before you begin the data collection.

REFERENCES

1. Winer, B. J. 1971. *Statistical principles in experimental design.* New York: McGraw-Hill.

2. Mendenhall, W. 1968. *Introduction to linear models and the design and analysis of experiments.* Belmont, Calif.: Wadsworth.

3. Kleinbaum, D. G., and Kupper, L. L. 1978. *Applied regression analysis and other multivariable methods.* North Scituate, Mass.: Duxbury.

4. John, P. W. M. 1971. *Statistical design and analysis of experiments.* New York: Macmillan. Pp. 120–121.

5. Williams, E. J. 1949. Experimental designs balanced for the estimation of residual effects of treatments. *Australian Journal of Scientific Research* Ser. A, 2: 149–168.

6. Williams, E. J. 1950. Experimental designs balanced for pairs of residual effects. *Australian Journal of Scientific Research* Ser. A, 3: 351–363.

7. Roethlisberger, F. J., and Dickson, W. I. 1939. *Management and the worker.* Cambridge, Mass.: Harvard University Press.

8. Homans, G. C. 1951. *The human group.* London: Routledge and Kegan Paul.

9. Landsberger, H. A. 1958. *Hawthorne revisited.* New York: Cornell University.

10. Blum, M. L. 1956. *Industrial psychology and its social foundations.* New York: Harper.

11. Miller, D. C., and Form, W. H. 1951. *Industrial sociology: An introduction to the sociology of work relations.* New York: Harper.

12. Mathe, G. 1973. Clinical examination of drugs. A scientific and ethical challenge. *Biomedicine* 18: 169–172.

13. Gehan, E. A., and Freireich, E. J. 1974. Non-randomized controls in cancer clinical trials. *New England Journal of Medicine* 290: 198–203.

14. Zelen, M. 1974. The randomization and stratification of patients to clinical trials. *Journal of Chronic Diseases* 27: 365–375.

15. Weinstein, M. C. 1974. Allocation of subjects in medical experiments. *New England Journal of Medicine* 291: 1278–1285.

16. Byar, D. P., *et al.* 1976. Randomized clinical trials: Perspectives on some recent ideas. *New England Journal of Medicine* 295: 74–80.

17. Peto, R., *et al.* 1976. Design and analysis of randomized clinical trials requiring prolonged observation of each patient: Introduction and design. *British Journal of Cancer* 34: 585–612.

18. Peto, R., *et al.* 1977. Design and analysis of randomized clinical trials requiring prolonged observation of each patient: Analysis and examples. *British Journal of Cancer* 35: 1–39.

19. Marks, R. *Analyzing Research Data.* Belmont, Calif.: Lifetime Learning Publications.

APPENDIX **A**

Review of Design Considerations

Before proceeding to the next phase of your research project, it is important to review your research design to make sure that all the decisions that have been made appear reasonable and acceptable now that the design is tentatively complete. To evaluate the experimental design, answer the following questions, which are merely a collection of the questions we have been asking at the ends of chapters all along.

I. What is the objective of this research project?

II. For this project, define the following terms and answer the questions.
   A. Universe
   B. Experimental unit
   C. Response variable(s)
   D. Factors
      1. Which are qualitative and which are quantitative?
      2. Which are observational and which are experimental?
      3. Which are extraneous factors?
      4. What are the levels for each factor defined?
   E. Is this project prospective or retrospective?
   F. Is this study experimental, case control, or a cross-sectional survey?

III. Choosing the response variable
   A. What are some appropriate response variables for this project?
   B. Which of these response variables will allow me to achieve the objective of this project?

C. Which of these response variables most objectively measure the phenomenon that I wish to study?
D. Which of these response variables can I realistically expect to collect with the resources available?
E. For each response variable to be measured, what is its type: nominal, ordinal, discrete, or continuous?

IV. Will repeated measures or blocking be used in the research project?
A. Is a repeated measure design, blocking, or matching physically possible for this project?
B. If repeated measures or blocking is possible, will additional information be gained? (Or, is there a basic difference in the response variable between experimental units in the absence of any factors?)
C. If repeated measures or blocking is employed, is it complete or incomplete? (Evaluate each factor separately.)

V. Choosing the sampling scheme
A. Which type of sampling scheme (random, stratified, cluster, or systematic) is most appropriate for my research project? Should a combination of methods be used?
B. Is it possible to employ the most appropriate sampling scheme?
C. Will the sample of experimental units that I choose using the chosen sampling scheme be representative of the entire universe?
D. What biases may be present in the sample?
E. If biases are present, how may they affect the conclusions that will be drawn?

VI. Choosing the sample size
A. If the chosen response variable is discrete or continuous, how much variability is expected between individual response variable measurements? If this quantity is unknown, what is the range of measurements?
B. What type of inference will I make, estimation or hypothesis testing?
C. How great an effect is to be shown (that is, how accurate an estimate, how large a difference between levels of a factor, etc.)?
D. What is the confidence coefficient for my estimation inference? What are α and β for my hypothesis-testing inference?
E. From a practical viewpoint, how large a sample can be taken?

VII. Choosing the randomization technique for assigning the levels of experimental factors to experimental units
A. Identify the experimental and extraneous factors from II.D. above
B. What are the potential extraneous factors for which I must control?
C. Will repeated measures or blocking be employed (that is, will the individual experimental units or groups of homogeneous experimental units receive more than one factor level combination of the experimental factors)?
D. What randomization technique shall I use to assign the levels of the experimental factors to the experimental units?

E. Should blinding (or masking) of either the experimental units or the researcher be employed?
F. Are there any moral or ethical considerations that should be weighed against the chosen randomization technique?
G. Is it necessary to obtain approval for the use of human subjects? If so, has the approval been given?

If you are satisfied with your responses to these questions, you are ready to begin considering the statistical analysis aspects of the research project.

Index

Boldface page numbers indicate pages where terms are defined.